The Amazing Language of Medicine

Robert B. Taylor

The Amazing Language of Medicine

Understanding Medical Terms and Their Backstories

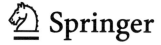 Springer

Robert B. Taylor, MD
Professor Emeritus
Department of Family Medicine
Oregon Health & Science University
School of Medicine
Portland, OR, USA

Professor
Department of Family and Community Medicine
Eastern Virginia Medical School
Norfolk, VA, USA

ISBN 978-3-319-50327-1   ISBN 978-3-319-50328-8   (eBook)
DOI 10.1007/978-3-319-50328-8

Library of Congress Control Number: 2016962313

This Springer imprint is published by Springer Nature
The registered company is Springer International Publishing AG
The registered company address is: Gewerbestrasse 11, 6330 Cham, Switzerland

Language is the house of Being. In its home man dwells. Those who think and those who create with words are the guardians of this home.

—Martin Heidegger. Letter on Humanism. London: Routledge; 1947, p. 217.

Preface

Words are, of course, the most powerful drug used by mankind.

—Rudyard Kipling [1]

Kipling goes on to say, "Not only do words infect, egotize, narcotize, and paralyze, but they enter into and colour the minutest cells of the brain..." [1]. Should we health professionals not know the full meanings and the sources of our medical words and phrases, these "powerful drugs" we all use each day?

If you want to know the full meaning of a word, the connotation as well as the dictionary definition, you need to know how the term arose. Every word in the medical dictionary came from somewhere. *Gracilis* is the Latin word for "slender" and today is the name of a long, thin muscle in the lower extremity. The word venereal comes from Venus, the Roman goddess of love. Knowing that *stoma* is the Greek word for mouth helps better understand diverse terms such as stomatitis and colostomy. In a sense, a word's story helps explain its aura.

The words we use in medicine—and in everyday life—did not enter our language wholly formed, like the goddess Athena sprang, as a grown adult and in full armor, from the head of Zeus. Consider that every word in the previous sentence came from somewhere, some source. The word "medicine," for example, can be traced back to the Latin word *medicina*, meaning the art of healing or a remedy. "Language" comes from the Latin *lingua*, meaning tongue. The name of "Zeus," chief among the ancient Greek gods, probably came from a pre-Hellenic language.

Most of today's medical terms had their origins in ancient Greek or Latin or perhaps other languages such as Quechua (quinine), Malay/Indonesian (agar), and Singhalese (beriberi). Some can be traced to very early times. Medical words may arise because of a sound (as in "cough"), an appearance or shape (think of the trapezius muscle), a region (Caucasian), a mythological figure (from Hygeia, the daughter Aesculapius, comes our word hygiene), or even a person's name (such as Hippocratic or Addisonian).

What was the source of the word syphilis? Why is a period of confinement to avoid the spread of communicable disease called quarantine? How did the drugs warfarin and nystatin get their names? What diseases have eponymic designations that relate to the patients affected rather than to the clinicians who described the ailments? What is a parachute research study? Why is the disease name gonorrhea actually a misnomer? If these questions seem intriguing, this is the book for you.

In a sense this is also a medical history book, tracing the often-meandering paths of words leading to our use today in the office, hospital, and laboratory. This book is not an etymologic dictionary, with words listed alphabetically and with aspirations to cover as many terms as pages allow; today, most of these notations are found online. It is also not a primer of medical terminology. In the pages to come, I present a series of tales about words that have intriguing backstories; the others I have left to dictionaries.

In discussing the words selected, I have tried to go beyond the usual brief explanations found in etymologic dictionaries. For example, the word atropine comes from Greek roots *a*, meaning "not," and *tropos*, meaning "to turn." But the tale is more complicated than just a word root with a prefix. It involves three Greek goddesses, the thread of life, and a potentially poisonous naturally occurring alkaloid— all described in Chap. 2.

As I have done in my other recent books, I use two types of reference listings. The first is the traditional list at the end of each chapter, with numbered citations in the text where I think the reader may want to follow a trail to its source. The other method is a reference to a specific page in one of the many book sources listed in the bibliography.

This book is written for all who provide health care to patients, who teach future health professionals, and who perform research that will make tomorrow's health care even better. By learning about *The Amazing Language of Medicine*, all of these professionals will have a richer appreciation of what they do each day.

Virginia Beach, VA, USA   Robert B. Taylor

Reference

1. Kipling R. Speech to the Royal College of Surgeons. London; 1923.

Contents

List of Figures

Chapter 1
About Medical Words and Their Origins

We health professionals speak an arcane language, often inscrutable to the uniniti-ated. I realized this recently when a neighbor brought me a report from her doctor, a document containing terms like sclerosis, dextroscoliosis, and white matter. She was flummoxed by the clinical argot and concerned that she had some serious dis-ease. I was able to translate the report into plain English and reassure her that what she had was more or less consistent with her age of 93. But in doing so, I felt a little like Samoset, translating for the Pilgrims of Plymouth Colony as they disembarked the Mayflower to share land with Native Americans in 1620.

The language of medicine is more or less English, but it is a very specialized subset of English, a sort of scholarly jargon. There are classical allusions, meta-phors, similes, eponyms, acronyms, authorisms, and honorisms. And our clinical dialect can, to patients and their families, be mysterious and often fearful. It cer-tainly can be confusing, with some persons believing, for instance, that hyperten-sion is a synonym for anxiety.

For those of us in the health profession, knowing word histories can help us use terms precisely. When I wonder about the sense of a word, I find it useful to look up the original meaning. Think about the **acetabulum**. The word comes from a Latin word meaning "vinegar cup," and I can visualize the cup shaped socket in the hip-bone that receives the head of the femur (Fig. 1.1). What's more, this bony structure shares a Latin root—*acetum*—with acetic acid, the main component, apart from water, of household vinegar. **Delirium** is not the same as dementia; perhaps this is a little easier to remember when knowing that the word delirium comes from Latin words that mean "plowing out of the furrows," suggesting a befuddled farmer dig-ging erratic troughs across his field. **Dementia**, on the other hand, means "out of one's mind," connoting memory loss and cognitive deficits.

Knowing a word's history helps us understand not only what it means but also how it got its current meaning, including some of its subtle connotative aspects. Shipley writes, "To know the origin of words is to know how men [and women] think, how they have fashioned their civilization. Word history traces the path of human fellowship, the bridges from mind to mind, from nation to nation" (Preface,

© Springer International Publishing AG 2017
R.B. Taylor, *The Amazing Language of Medicine*,
DOI 10.1007/978-3-319-50328-8_1

Fig. 1.1 The hip socket/acetabulum. Credit: Pearson Scott Foresman. Public Domain https:// commons.wikimedia.org/ wiki/File:Socket_1_(PSF). png

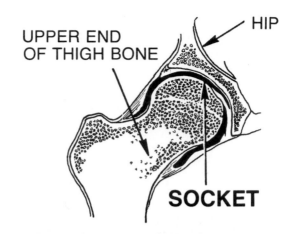

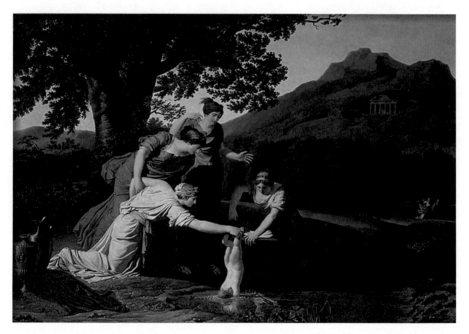

Fig. 1.2 Thetis dipping the infant Achilles in the River Styx. By: Antoine Borel (1743–1810). Public Domain https://commons.wikimedia.org/wiki/File:Thetis_Immerses_Son_Achilles_in_Water_of_River_Styx_by_Antoine_Borel.jpg

p. vii). We modern clinicians describe the calcaneal tendon (connecting the gastrocnemius and soleus muscles to the tuberosity of the calcaneus) as the **Achilles tendon,** an eponym that has persisted for centuries. Those with a liberal arts education will recognize the tale of how the nymph Thetis, the mother of the Greek hero Achilles, dipped him as an infant into the River Styx, holding him by the heel (Fig. 1.2). This dunking made him invulnerable to injury except in the one site that had not been submerged, exactly where an arrow from the bow of Paris struck and killed him during the Trojan War. The tendon did not receive the sobriquet Achilles until so named in 1693 by Dutch anatomist Philip Verheyen (1648–1710), after he had dissected his own amputated leg. The clinical nuance of the eponym is not just the anatomical connection between muscle and bone; it is that the Achilles tendon is a site of *vulnerability*—the so-called Achilles heel—as any victim of an Achilles tendon rupture will attest.

Here is an amusing anecdote about a tendon injury: In 1907, Australian dancer Victor Goulet ruptured his Achilles tendon. Surgeons replaced his damaged tendon with a transplant from a wallaby [1]. We can only imagine the changes to the course of medical history if the word wallaby were to supplant Achilles in discussion of either the tendon or the heel.

Some Words About the Medical Words We Use Today

The histories of some of our words are quite lengthy, indeed. For example, according to researchers at Reading University in the United Kingdom, the words **I**, **we**, **two**, and **three** date back many millennia, perhaps as much as 40,000 years. According to Professor Mark Pagel, "The sounds used to make these words would have been used by all speakers of the Indo-European languages throughout history." [2] The word **one** is slightly younger, while **four**, in English at least, is a relative newcomer.

The Indo-European languages cited by Pagel, and from which today's English is descended, are a family of communication systems derived from the prehistoric Proto-Indo-European family of languages. Thus English shares a common ancestry with such diverse modern tongues as Persian, Hindi, Catalan, Yiddish, Polish, and several dozen others.

What about medical words as a subset of modern English? The latest edition of *Dorland's Illustrated Medical Dictionary* describes more than 120,000 medical terms in its 2176 pages. It weighs 8.2 pounds [3]. The source of most of the words described is ancient Greek or Latin. In what I consider a heroic exercise in scholarship, Butler catalogued more than 50,000 words in the 24th edition of *Dorland's Illustrated Medical Dictionary*. The author found that Greek was the source of 58.5%, and 21.8% came from Latin. Some combination words had roots that came from both Greek and Latin, and in some cases, the Greek or Latin roots are combined with another language. Only a few medical terms, 2.9%, came to us from English [4]. Most of these, of course, can be traced to words of the earlier Indo-European languages.

How many new words does a student learn in the 4 years of medical school? There is no precise answer to this question, but one author has gone out on a limb, estimating that the average college graduate has a vocabulary of some 15,000 words and adds another 15,000 words during medical school education. That calculates to 3750 words per year, approximately ten new words each day [5].

My Interest in Words

In medical school, whenever I encountered a new word, I looked up the derivation and recorded this in my notebook. I have continued my fascination with words and have acquired many more than my share of books about word origins, especially those that tell the beginnings of medical terms. The evidence of this assertion lies in the bibliography at the end of this book. The field of knowledge that is concerned with word derivations is **etymology**, this word itself coming from two ancient Greek words meaning the study of the true sense of a word.

Ancient Greek and Latin are considered "completed languages" in that they are no longer evolving; existing words are not modified and new words are not coined. This is significant because most of today's medical terms come from these early languages and hence are "carved in stone." The **deltoid** muscle takes its name from the triangular shape of the Greek letter *delta*. Latin has given us, directly assimilated into our medical vocabulary, *stapes* (stirrup) and *cervix* (neck). None of these terms will change. In contrast English, French, Spanish, and other modern languages are "incomplete"; that is, they are constantly changing. In 2009, the English language reached a milestone when **web 2.0**, meaning the second generation of web development, was designated the millionth word in the English language.

Words, including those used by health care professionals, are actually living things. Words have personalities. Each word has appeal or lack of it, status, and ancestry. Words also mate, yielding progeny—neologisms formed by linking word roots and other parts. Combining syllables with distinct meanings has given us thousands of what were once medical neologisms. Consider **hyperlipidemia** (elevated + fats + blood), **dermatitis** (skin + inflammation of), and **etiology** (cause + to speak of).

Some medical words are pleasing: a few of my favorites are *borborygmus, murmur*, and *serendipity* (the latter often applied to scientific discoveries). I am also partial to *onomatopoeia*, used in the title of Chap. 6. Hendrickson [6] reports that American poet Carl Sandburg (1878–1967) was partial to *Monongahela*, while Irish author James Joyce (1882–1941) favored *cuspidor. Alabaster* was among the favorite words of British philosopher Bertrand Russell (1872–1970). My vote goes to **Monongahela**, the name of a river in southwestern Pennsylvania, one of America's few rivers that flow from south to north, and the name of a small city on the west bank of this river. But I may have a slight bias, because I grew up in the town of Monongahela, Pennsylvania.

On the other hand, there are some unpleasant-sounding words in medicine. Examples include **flatulent, grippe**, and **scabies. Scatological** is an ugly word; **moron** is mean. In fact, Pagel predicts that before too many decades have passed, some words—such as **dirty, guts, wipe**, and **stab**—will pass into lexicographic oblivion, having been replaced with more euphonious synonyms [2].

Clearly words, including medical words, have social status. In ancient Rome, there were the patricians (upper class) and the plebeians (commoners). If they were alive today and speaking English, the patricians would say **perspire, expectorate, abdomen**, and **underarm**. The plebeians would use the words **sweat, spit, belly**, and **armpit**.

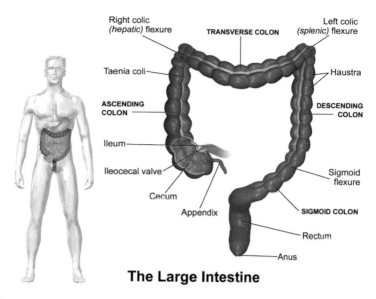

The Large Intestine

Fig. 1.3 The human colon, a hollow viscus. Source: Blausen.com staff. "Blausen gallery 2014." *Wikiversity Journal of Medicine.* Public Domain DOI:10.15347/wjm/2014.010. ISSN 20018·762 https://commons.wikimedia.org/wiki/File:Blausen_0604_LargeIntestine2.png

Every word has a distinct, and sometimes colorful, origin. **Monongahela**, for example, comes from a Native American language and means "river of falling banks." Words that have come to us from the ancient Greeks include **phalanx** (line of soldiers), **pylorus** (gatekeeper), and **colon** (hollow) (Fig. 1.3). From Latin, we get **dura mater** (tough mother), and **vagus** (wandering) is the name of the seemingly peripatetic tenth cranial nerve. **Flatus** describes a puff of wind in Latin. Nonclassical languages have given us many medical words, such as **cascara** (a plant with laxative properties, Spanish), **tsutsugamushi** (dangerous bug, Japanese), and **agar** (a gelatinous substance derived from seaweed, Malay). And some of today's medical terms have followed a long and tortuous path. As an example, the word **quinsy**, indicating a severe and perhaps obstructing throat infection, began in ancient Greek as *kynanchein*, meaning to choke a dog. The word was adapted into Latin as *quinancia*, to strangle. It then became *qwinaci* in Old French and later **quinsy** in English.

Thus ends the etymology lesson. The next nine chapters in the book are more about descriptive narratives than etymologic lexicography.

What's Ahead?

In Chap. 2, I will describe some classical myths and heroic figures that have found their way into our medical vocabulary: the antics of Pan, the curse of Ondine, and the allure of Aphrodite.

Chapter 3 covers tales of many descriptive terms we use, including activities, occupations, customs, and appearances. Here I will tell about our use of the words nausea, rabies, carotid, and digitalis.

Although most medical words come to us from (or through) Greek and Latin, other languages have contributed to our current clinical lexicon. Sources include not only the Indo-European languages other than Greek or Latin. We also use words that have come from Asian, South American, Pacific Island, Arabic, and other tongues. Examples found in Chap. 4 include quinine, alcohol, triage, and bezoar.

Colchicine, ammonia, magnesia, and plaster of Paris all were named for places, although some took some fascinating turns through history, as described in Chap. 5.

Chapter 6 is about metaphors, similes, and echoic words—what something looks like or sounds like—and how these words happened to emerge and survive. Examples include pica, mitral, ether, and whooping cough.

The medical dictionary is rich with the names of science's and medicine's giants and a few who just happened to be the beneficiaries of serendipitous discoveries (to use one of my favorite words here). Chapter 7 tells stories you may not know about the Circle of Willis, Huntington chorea, and Christmas disease.

Chapter 8 presents authorisms—neologisms that can be attributed to an individual, often with an appealing story behind the word's creation. Who first gave us the words tonic, streptococcus, anaphylaxis, angina pectoris, and the longest word in the English language; and what are the accounts surrounding these invented words?

All the medical terms in this book have origins that are interesting somehow. Chapter 9 tells of some that are especially intriguing. How does heaven relate to the origin of the word influenza? How did the innominate artery get its name? What architectural feature inspired the creation of the term fornicate? And what is the story behind the Kochleffel syndrome?

In Chap. 10, I present some word derivations that are confusing or controversial. If Charles Dickens' character Mr. Pickwick was not the namesake of the Pickwickian syndrome, who was? Does caesarean have anything to do with Roman emperor Julius Caesar? What are the fundamental misconceptions in the origin of the terms gonorrhea, artery, hysteria, and essential hypertension?

Any book on word origins is essentially a history book. And, astonishing as it may seem, historians often disagree on what happened way back when. So, in this book, when controversy exists—such as the origin of the terms barbiturate, condom, and Saint Anthony's fire—I will present what I believe the most plausible story, but often with some qualification to indicate that not all agree with the version presented.

The amazing language of medicine is also still expanding. New words are being added every day. Consider the term **iPatient**, coined by Abraham Verghese, describing "the chart as surrogate for the patient." Verghese goes on to say, "iPatients are handily discussed in the bunker, while the real patients keep the beds warm and ensure that the folders bearing their names stay alive on the computer" [7]. Other new terms recently introduced into our vocabulary are **diabesity, metabolic syndrome, telehealth**, and a host of new drug names. *Dorland's Illustrated*

Medical Dictionary, 32nd edition [3], contains several thousand new words. Today's medical language is far from "completed."

Because I consulted print reference sources at many times during manuscript preparation, there is a bibliography detailing word origin, medical history, and other books cited on the pages to come. As mentioned in the preface, I have cited these sources repeatedly, providing page numbers for those who would like to consult original sources. In addition, there are selected references in each chapter for key facts from the current literature and the Internet.

Here is full disclosure about my presentation of word roots. I am a physician with an interest in word origins and medical history, and I like a good story. I am not a Greek or Latin expert, despite my 2 years of high school Latin and the earnest efforts of my literature professors at Bucknell University to make me a classical scholar. For these reasons, and because this book does not aspire to be an etymologic dictionary, Latin and other word roots are sometimes specifically identified (such as *stapes* and *cervix*, above) and at other times simply described. And because few of us today can recite the Greek alphabet, the ancient Greek word roots discussed are not presented in the alphabet of Hippocrates and Plato.

At this point, it is time to turn the page, literally going back in (word) history and begin to enjoy the stories behind some of the medical terms we use today.

References

1. Lloyd J, Mitchinson J, Harkin J. 1,141 Quite interesting facts to knock you sideways. New York: W. W. Norton and Company; 2015.
2. Oldest English words identified. BBC News, Feb. 26, 2009. Available at: http://news.bbc.co.uk/2/hi/uk/7911645.stm#
3. Dorland's Illustrated Medical Dictionary, 32nd ed. Philadelphia: Saunders; 2011.
4. Butler RF. Sources of the medical vocabulary. J Med Educ. 1980;55:128.
5. Joh JW. Approximately how many terms does a 1st or 2nd year medical student memorize per weekday?Quora.Availableat:https://www.quora.com/Approximately-how-many-terms-does-a-1st-or-2nd-year-medical-student-memorize-per-weekday
6. Hendrickson R. The literary life and other curiosities. New York: Viking; 1981, p. 336.
7. Verghese A. Culture shock—patient as icon, icon as patient. N Engl J Med. 2008;359:2748.

Chapter 2
Medical Words with Mythological Origins

During my college years, on my way to medical school, I became intrigued with the Greek gods Apollo, Athena, Hercules, Atlas, Aphrodite, and all the rest. I made an earnest effort to learn about them, including the various family trees. I discovered that, first of all, there are a lot of Greek (and Roman) gods. And, second, they were both promiscuous and fecund. The gods did not seem to care whether they or their consorts were married or not. Apollo bedded with more than 60 women—among them Daphne, Cassandra, and Coronis—and sired scores of children, including Aesculapius, the god of medicine. The gods mated with other gods, nymphs, and mortals. For example, Coronis, mother of Aesculapius, was a mortal. Zeus had more than 90 children with some 70 women, both divine and mortal. Apollo also had several male partners. Aphrodite enjoyed a number of consorts, including Poseidon, Dionysus, and Zeus.

When the Romans conquered Greece, they assimilated much of their culture, including their gods. But they changed many of the names: Aphrodite, goddess of love, beauty, and sexuality, became Venus. Hermes came to be known as Mercury, Zeus became Jupiter, Hera was renamed Juno, and Poseidon was called Neptune by the Romans.

All this is important to us because the names of Greek and Roman gods are scattered throughout the medical dictionary. Just a few examples are **Hymen**, the god of marriage; **Proteus**, the sea god; **Psyche**, goddess of the human soul; and **Mercury**, the messenger god whose name is attached to both a planet and an element. All of these will be described shortly. This chapter tells stories of how we health-care professionals came to use so many words that began with myths arising some 2500 years ago.

In the Grove of Academia

This book being an academic effort, and with many health professionals working in academic medical centers, it seems appropriate to begin our chapter with the story of the mythological figure whose name led to our current word **academia** and hence

© Springer International Publishing AG 2017
R.B. Taylor, *The Amazing Language of Medicine*,
DOI 10.1007/978-3-319-50328-8_2

Fig. 2.1 Helen of Troy. By
Evelyn de Morgan, 1898.
Public domain. https://
commons.wikimedia.org/
wiki/File:Helen_of_Troy.jpg

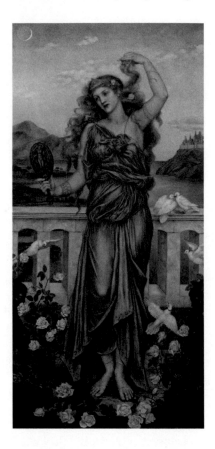

academic. Our tale begins with the Trojan War, chronicled in Homer's *Iliad* and
other sources.

The most beautiful woman in the world, Helen of Troy, was the daughter of Zeus
and Leda, queen of Sparta, and the sister of Pollux, Castor, and Clytemnestra
(Fig. 2.1). When she was a 12-year-old girl, Helen was kidnapped by Theseus, the
mythical king of Athens. A Greek youth named Academus told her older twin brothers where Helen had been hidden, allowing them to rescue their sister. Later, according to the words of English playwright Christopher Marlowe (1564–1593) in *Doctor
Faustus*, Helen would become "the face that launched a thousand ships."

The grateful Spartans rewarded Academus with an olive grove at a site near
Athens. Eventually this land became a public park. Then, in the fourth century BCE,
the philosopher Plato began a school of philosophy in the Grove of Academus,
teaching students as he walked among the olive trees. The school of philosophy
came to be called the **Academia**.

Through Roman times and later, the word **academy** came to describe any institu-
tion of higher learning, whether philosophy, medicine, or economics. English poet

John Milton (1608–1674) popularized the phrase "groves of Academe" in his poem *Paradise Regained*:

> The olive groves of Academe,
> Plato's retirement, where the Attic bird
> Trills her thick-warbl'd notes the summer long.

Following his death, Plato was buried near the Grove of Academus. And we inherited the words **academe, academia,** and **academic.**

The Odd Origin of Apollo Disease

Yes, there is an Apollo disease of the ocular conjunctiva, but most of us in the developed world have not seen a case. How did an eye disease come to be named for the Greek god Apollo?

Apollo, son of Zeus and Leto, had a diverse portfolio. He was the god of sun, light, music, prophecy, poetry, and more. He dispatched arrows that could bring plague to his enemies, and he was also the chief god of healing.

The Apollo space program—Project Apollo   was the third such program carried out by the United States National Aeronautics and Space Administration (NASA); the previous program was named Project Mercury. The first Apollo flight was in 1968, and in July 1969, astronauts Neil Armstrong and Buzz Aldrin exited the Apollo 11 spaceship and walked on the moon (Fig. 2.2). And, more pertinent to our story, when they returned to Earth, they brought with them lunar rock and soil samples. Their achievement was known and praised around the world.

Our story now moves to the nation of Ghana in West Africa. It was here that, in 1969, there developed a new pandemic of hemorrhagic conjunctivitis of the eyes caused by an enterovirus [1]. Believing that the disease had been brought to Earth with soil samples from the moon, the local people called it "Apollo 11 disease." We don't even know if the person who first coined the sobriquet knew of the Greek god, but in 1969, everyone knew of Apollo 11. Over time, the "11" disappeared, and the conjunctival infection came to be simply **Apollo disease.** The conjunctivitis is a benign infection, with recovery generally occurring in a few weeks. But the disease name has stuck, and the eponymous disease designation is unrelated to the Greek deity being a healer.

Mercury and its Movements

Mercury is the Roman name of the Greek god Hermes, the messenger of the gods with special duties in regard to commerce, travelers, and thieves. Considered to be swift in his movements, he is typically pictured as having winged sandals.

Fig. 2.2 Astronaut Buzz
Aldrin, lunar module pilot,
stands on the surface of the
moon near the leg of the
lunar module, *Eagle*,
during the Apollo 11
moonwalk. Astronaut Neil
Armstrong, mission
commander, took this
photograph. Source:
National Aeronautics and
Space Administration.
Public Domain. https://
commons.wikimedia.org/
wiki/File:Aldrin_
Apollo_11_original.jpg

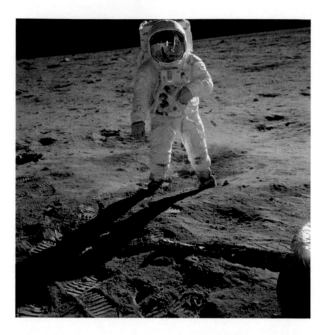

In the third millennium BCE, the Sumerians knew of the celestial body we now call Mercury, the fastest-moving planet in the solar system. Because of its speed, the Greeks named it for Hermes, later changed to Mercury when the Romans co-opted the Greek gods under new names.

This brings us to the element with atomic number 80 and the symbol Hg. How did this metal come to share its name with a Roman god and a planet? The clue is the element's nickname: **quicksilver**. Mercury's chemical symbol is Hg, coming from the Greek word *hydrargyrum*, meaning liquid silver (Fig. 2.3). The material may be a metal, but it moves; it doesn't just sit there like copper or zinc. It is a liquid at room temperature. It may not move very quickly, but it was the metal's ability to move at all that prompted it to be named for the swiftest of the Greek gods and the most rapidly moving planet.

Mercury has a long and colorful history in medical therapeutics and in toxicology. Mercury was famously the first (more or less) effective treatment for syphilis. Its use began in the sixteenth century, not long after the disease first spread across Europe. To treat the "great pox," mercury was consumed as an elixir, applied as an ointment, or inhaled as fumes. Treatment might continue for years, leading to the popular saying, "An evening with Venus; a lifetime with Mercury."

Side effects of mercury therapy included oral ulcers, neuropathies, and renal failure. Yet the treatment continued to be used until supplanted by Salvarsan, an arsenical compound developed by German scientist Paul Ehrlich (1854–1915) in 1910.

There is a colorful historic footnote to the legacy of Lewis and Clark in their expedition to explore the Louisiana Purchase in 1804 and 1805. As they planned for the trip west, the leaders recognized two things: First, there would be no physician

Fig. 2.3 Drops of liquid mercury. Source: Unkky. Creative Commons. https://commons.wikimedia.org/wiki/File:Billes-Hg.jpg

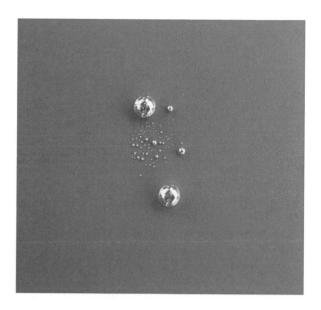

in their group, and, second, the anticipated diet of game meat and few vegetables foretold of constipation problems. Luckily, there was a powerful remedy at the time. It was *Dr. Rush's Bilious Pills*, created by Dr. Benjamin Rush, a leading physician of the day and a signer of the Declaration of Independence. Before departing on their journey, the explorers stocked their medicine kit with a large supply of these pills, which they called *Thunderclappers*; the active ingredient was mercurous chloride, a powerful purgative. We know this today because traces of mercury can still be found in the soil of sites where the Corps of Discovery camped.

As we come to the twentieth century, during my early practice years and before the days of furosemide (Lasix), we physicians administered an injectable drug called mercuhydrin when the patient experienced edema that needed to be treated. This was the brand name of a mercury compound that caused a brisk diuresis by poisoning the kidney.

This brings me to the toxicity of mercury. Brain damage resulted from the use of mercury-containing products that were absorbed by milliners who made felt hats in the eighteenth and nineteenth centuries. The Japanese city of Minamata became famous in 1956 when it was found that the discharge of mercury-containing toxic waste into the bay was being accumulated in seafood that was the staple component of the local diet. The result was a syndrome with neurologic abnormalities, convulsions, coma, and often death—what we now call **Minamata disease**.

Mercury poisoning still occurs occasionally. Although the etiology has been disputed, in 2008, actor Jeremy Piven quit his role in a Broadway play, citing symptoms of weakness and dizziness, attributed to **mercury toxicity** when high levels were found in his blood. Piven attributes the high blood mercury level to a very high intake of sushi in his diet [2].

Atlas and the Celestial Globe

Atlas is the name of the first cervical vertebra, the one that supports the head. The bone was so named by Italian anatomist Andreas Vesalius (1514–1564), as an allusion to the Greek god of the same name.

Atlas, one of the Titans, was the god of astronomy and navigation. After being on the losing side in the war of the Titans against Olympians, Atlas was punished by Zeus by commanding him to bear the weight of the heavens upon his shoulders. Yes, Atlas holds up the sky, not the Earth, as commonly believed (Fig. 2.4).

The spot where Zeus commanded Atlas to stand was the western edge of the Earth, at least as known by the ancient Greeks. Somewhere in this area was a large body of water. It was only appropriate to name vast sea after the Titan—the Atlantic Ocean. And the mythical civilization beneath the body of water was eponymously also named Atlantis.

Today, if you ask a schoolchild what Atlas holds on his shoulders, the answer is likely to be the "world" or "Earth" and not the heavens. Contributing to this misunderstanding about Atlas' burden is a widely disseminated book of maps by Flemish geographer Gerardus Mercator (1512–1594) (Evans, p. 57). The cover of the book showed an image of Atlas holding the world, not the sky, and from that seminal book, we now call a collection of maps an "atlas."

Aphrodite Arising from the Sea

Aphrodite was the Greek goddess of beauty, love, and procreation. There are conflicting stories of her birth. In one she is the daughter of Zeus and the Earth goddess, Dione. In another tale, she arose from the sea foam, floating ashore in a scallop shell. In fact, the source of the name Aphrodite is the Greek word *aphros*, meaning "foam."

Whatever her origin, Aphrodite seemed to have no childhood, being born fully mature and remarkably desirable. Her chief consort was Adonis, but she was less than faithful to him. She had a number of sexual conquests, including Hermes, messenger of the gods; Poseidon, god of the sea; and Dionysus, god of the vine and winemaking. From the goddess' abundant sexuality and her willingness to share her favors obligingly, we get the word **aphrodisiac**, referring to something that causes sexual desire.

History has many instances of the quest for the ideal love potion. In Shakespeare's *A Midsummer Night's Dream* (II, i), Oberon seeks a magical aphrodisiac:

Fetch me that flower; the herb I showed thee once:
The juice of it on a sleeping eyelid laid
Will make a man or woman madly dote
Upon the next live creature that it sees.

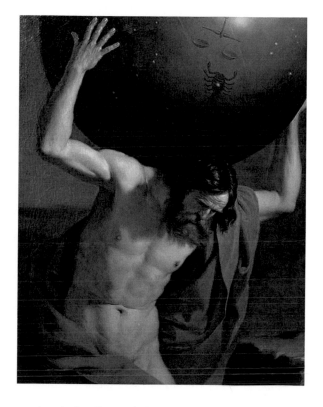

Fig. 2.4 Atlas holding up the celestial globe—not the planet Earth. By Guercinio (1591–1666). Public Domain. https://commons. wikimedia.org/wiki/ File:Atlas_holding_up_ the_celestial_globe_-_ Guercino_(1646).jpg

The story goes on. It seems that Aphrodite and Hermes had a two-sexed child named Hermaphroditus, merging the names of the parents. This mythological individual, generally depicted in classical art as a female with male genitalia, represented the state of being androgynous. Eventually Hermaphroditus fused with the nymph Salmacis, to become one body with features of both sexes, giving us our word **hermaphrodite** to describe someone with both male and female charactcristics.

The Romans embraced the concept of an attractive and sexually adventurous goddess, changing the name from Aphrodite to Venus. In Rome, she continued her amorous exploits, with a role in prenuptial rites. One legend holds that by being mother of Aeneas, who came to Italy when Troy fell to the Greeks, Aphrodite/Venus was mother to the Roman people. From her name, we have the word **venereal**.

Children of Aphrodite: Eros, Hymen, and Priapus

Aphrodite had several children who, all on their own, achieved eponymous renown. One was Hymen, her son by Dionysus, also known as Bacchus. Hymen was revered in Greece as the god of marriage. If Hymen did not attend one's marriage, the union was doomed. He is mentioned and praised by Cassandra in Euripides' *The Trojan Women*: "Oh Hymen, king of marriage! Blest is the bridegroom, blest am I also, a maiden soon to wed a princely lord in Argos." It is probably worth noting here that Cassandra describes herself as a "maiden." The word **hymen** meant "membrane" in ancient Greek, and today the "maidenhead" often has significance at the time of the wedding night.

Then there was Eros, son of Aphrodite, although his paternity is disputed—maybe Zeus, or Hermes, or Dionysus. We can see why classical mythology can be confusing. Eros was the Greek god of love and became Cupid in Roman times (Fig. 2.5). Eros meddled in the relationships between the gods, using his arrows to foster romantic, and often ill-advised, relationships. Roman poet Ovid (43 BCE-17 CE) wrote in *Metamorphosis 10*:

> Once, when Venus' son [Eros] was kissing her, his quiver dangling down, a jutting arrow, unbeknown, had grazed her breast. She pushed the boy away. In fact the wound was deeper than it seemed, though unperceived at first. [And she became] enraptured by the beauty of a man [Adonis].

From the name of this god, we have the word **erotic**. And from his chubby Roman counterpart, Cupid, we have **cupidity**, which somehow has metamorphosed from meaning "erotic desire" to the current definition of "desire for wealth."

Then there is Priapus, also a son of Dionysus and Aphrodite, who was the patron god of merchant seamen. Priapus is remembered today for his enormous phallus, perpetually turgid, depicted in classical paintings and sculpture. Several such images were found in the ruins of Pompeii and Herculaneum. In medicine today, we have the uncomfortable condition called **priapism**, the state that prompts the warning on phosphodiesterase inhibitor drugs to call your physician if you have an erection lasting four hours or longer.

Priapus spent his spare time with Pan, part man and part goat, god of shepherds and the wild, who was fond of playing his flute and chasing nymphs. His fearsome appearance and shrill voice frightened many. From his rambunctious behavior, Pan gave us the word **panic** (Onions, p. 646).

Children of Aesculapius

Until recent years, new physicians recited the Hippocratic oath, now largely replaced by the Declaration of Geneva. One of the several reasons that the Hippocratic oath has been declared anachronistic is its opening sentence:

> I swear by Apollo the physician, and Aesculapius the surgeon, likewise Hygieia and Panacea, and call all the gods and goddesses to witness, that I will observe and keep this underwritten oath, to the utmost of my power and judgment.

Modern physicians no longer swear by ancient mythological deities, not even Aesculapius, held by the Greeks to be the god of medicine, or Apollo, god of knowledge and health. But who were Hygieia and Panacea? They were among the several

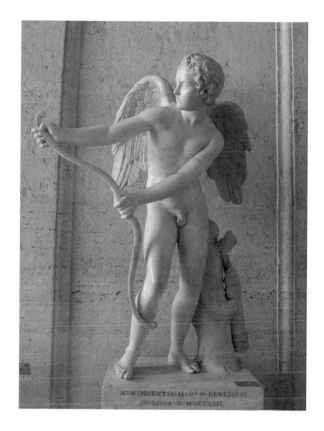

children of Aesculapius, five daughters and four sons, all of whom played roles in regard to health. Aceso, for example, was the goddess of healing, and Iaso was goddess of recovery from illness. But only two—Hygieia and Panacea—are mentioned in the Hippocratic oath. And only these two are the sources of medical terms we use today.

Hygeia was goddess of cleanliness and sanitation and was often portrayed in art and sculpture as a young woman drinking from a jug or feeding a large serpent that entwines her body, the latter depiction an example of the ancient Greek connection between snakes and health care. There were temples erected to Hygeia in Epidaurus, Corinth, Pergamon, and Cos, the latter the island home of Hippocrates. We have incorporated her name into the medical lexicon as **hygiene** (Pepper, p. 126). Perhaps the authors of the Hippocratic oath anticipated that sanitation would eventually save more lives worldwide than all the medicine and surgery physicians could muster over time.

Panacea, goddess of the universal cure, possessed a special remedy that relieved all ills. Our word **panacea**—a magic bullet for all diseases—comes directly from her name.

Atropine and the Three Fates

The mythological mistresses of destiny were the three Fates (Fig. 2.6), children of Zeus and Themis, whose name in Greek translates to mean "divine law." The youngest of the goddesses was Clotho, who spun the thread of human life and who was the source of our word **cloth**. She had wide-ranging powers over persons' lives and, incidentally, worked with Hermes to create the Greek alphabet.

The second sister was Lachesis, who measured the thread of life, determining the lifespan of each person. Although not represented in medical terminology, somehow Lachesis has come to be the name of a genus of pit vipers called bushmasters, found in Central and South America.

The third and oldest sister was Atropos, whose name comes from *a-*, meaning "not," and *tropos*, meaning "changeable"—the inflexible one. Often depicted holding shears, she determined how a person would die; she ended the days of each by cutting the thread of life. In medicine we have the highly toxic *Atropa belladonna*, or Deadly Nightshade, allegedly used by Livia to murder her husband, Roman Emperor Augustus (63 BCE–14 CE). And today we have the drug **atropine**, with a number of practical uses in medicine.

An extract of the roots of Deadly Nightshade was used to enlarge the pupils of would-be glamorous women in Renaissance Italy. The material used came to be called **belladonna**, from *bella* (fair, beautiful) and *donna* (lady). Of course, by using this drug, these lovelies could focus just about as well as we can today when our eyes are dilated for an ophthalmologic exam. An alternative theory for the etymology of **belladonna** is that the name arose because this chemical was what a famous killer of the time used to poison beautiful women.

The Sphinx and Muscles that Squeeze Tightly

Not all mythological word origins are related to Gods and Titans. There are also kings, shepherds, and other mortals, as well as monsters. One of the latter was the sphinx, a creatively fanciful ogre with the head of a woman and body of a lion (Fig. 2.7). It was presented as a gift by the goddess Hera to the Egyptian city of Thebes, where it stood at the city's front gates, challenging each arriving person with a riddle: "What moves on four legs in the morning, two at noon, and three in the evening?" Failure to answer correctly led to death.

Although the riddles are different, opera fans may see a parallel to the three riddles posed under threat of death that faced suitors of the beautiful heroine who gives the opera its name: *Turandot*.

The word sphinx comes from the Greek word *sphingo*, meaning "to squeeze." And those who failed to solve the riddle of the sphinx were, according to some legends, dispatched by strangulation. And the answer to the riddle is *man*, who crawls on four extremities as a baby, walks on two legs as an adult, and uses a cane in old age.

Fig. 2.6 The Triumph of Death, or The Three Fates. Flemish tapestry (probably Brussels, ca. 1510–1520). Public Domain. https://commons.wikimedia.org/wiki/File:The_Triumph_of_Death,_or_The_Three_Fates.jpg

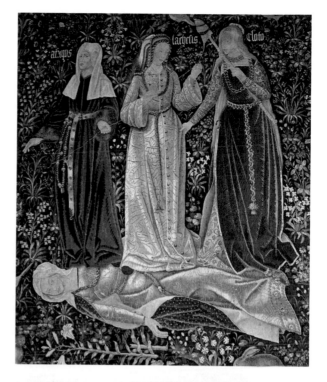

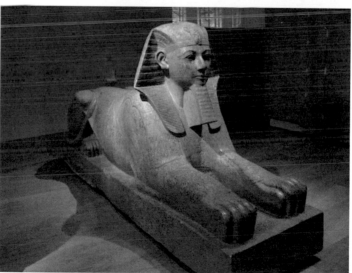

Fig. 2.7 Sphinx, Metropolitan Museum of Art, New York City. Source: Юкатан. Public Domain. https://commons.wikimedia.org/wiki/File:Sphinx_Metropolitan.jpg

Eventually one man solved the riddle. It was Oedipus, discussed next. The sphinx was so enraged by the correct response that it strangled itself to death. As a legacy we have the word to describe a muscle that contracts to control body fluids and gases: **sphincter**.

Oedipus and His Mother

We remember Oedipus, son of Laius and Jocasta, king and queen of Thebes, not only because he solved the riddle of the sphinx but also for his family misadventures.

When he was born, it was prophesied that Oedipus would kill his father and marry his mother. To avoid this fate, the child was sent out of the kingdom. Eventually, as a young man traveling to Thebes, Oedipus quarrels with a stranger on the road and kills him in a duel; that man, unknown to Oedipus, was his father. The young man continues his journey, arrives in Thebes, outwits the sphinx, and becomes king. He goes on to marry the now-widowed queen Jocasta, thus unwittingly wedding his own mother. It was apparently a fruitful marriage; they had four children together. When the truth is learned, Jocasta hangs herself and Oedipus gouges out his own eyes.

Sophocles, writing in the fifth century BCE, tells the story in *Oedipus Rex* (Oedipus the King). It awaited Sigmund Freud (1856–1939) (Fig. 2.8) to medicalize the legend as the **Oedipus complex** to describe a "family romance" (Garrison, p. 702). Curiously, the name Oedipus comes from Greek words meaning "swollen foot."

Narcissus, Echo, and an Ill-Fated Attraction

Here is another doomed mythological pair, described in Ovid's *Metamorphoses*. Echo was a chatty nymph, cursed by Hera, because of one of the all-too-common divine intrigues, to be able only to repeat the last words of others. She became a verbal mimic. The communication-challenged nymph falls in love with Narcissus, son of a river god, and prays to Aphrodite for help with her relationship. Aphrodite, however, jealous of Echo, causes the nymph to vanish, leaving only a disembodied voice, and the source of our word **echo**.

Narcissus, who had rudely spurned Echo's advances, was so attractive that he became enchanted with his own reflection in a pond, jumped in to reach the object of his desire, and drowned. When the nymphs came to his funeral, they found only a flower, now called by the self-absorbed lad's name, Narcissus (Fig. 2.9). The word **narcissism**, as a psychiatric state of excessive self-love, was enshrined in the medical literature in 1899 by German psychiatrist Paul Näcke (1851–1913) [3].

Fig. 2.8 Sigmund Freud, founder of psychoanalysis, 1922. By Max Halberstadt (1882–1940). Public Domain. https://commons. wikimedia.org/wiki/ File:Sigmund_Freud_ LIFE.jpg

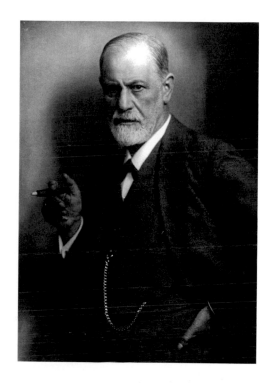

Fig. 2.9 Narcissus calcicola. By Olaf Lcillinger. Creative Commons. https:// commons.wikimedia.org/ wiki/File:Narcissus. calcicola.7114.jpg

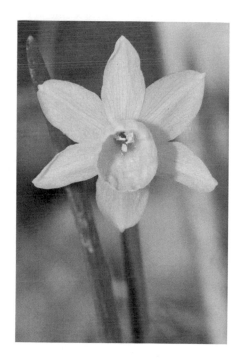

Undine and the Penalty for a Broken Promise

Paracelsus (1493–1541) wrote of Undine, also called Ondine, as the spirit of the waters, who was later incorporated into medieval German and Scandinavian folklore (Dirckx, p. 72). She was the central character of an 1811 novella titled *Undine* by Friedrich de la Motte Fouqué (Onions, p. 959). Here is the story.

Ondine was extraordinarily beautiful, but was born without a soul. She would, however, obtain a soul (and all the joys and pains of being human) if she married a mortal and had their child. She marries handsome Palemon, and, at their wedding, the bridegroom pledges, "My every waking breath will be my pledge of love and faithfulness to you." This proved to be a fateful choice of words.

Following the birth of their son, Ondine discovers Palemon in flagrante delicto with another woman. She curses her husband so that he will breathe normally while awake, but cease to breathe if he falls asleep. Eventually sleep overtook Palemon; lacking autonomic respiratory activity, he died for lack of oxygen. This has given rise to the eponymous **Ondine curse**, also known as idiopathic central alveolar hypoventilation. Patients with this rare disorder, like Palemon, fail to breathe during sleep and thus need nocturnal respiratory support.

The French Disease and the Shepherd

Not long after Christopher Columbus and his shipmates returned to Spain from their adventures, an apparently new disease spread rapidly across Europe. In 1494, the French laid siege to Naples, and during this battle, in a nefarious instance of biologic warfare, the Neapolitans sent diseased prostitutes to infect the French troops. The French troops and subsequent armies of conquest then helped spread the disease across Europe and Asia.

The disease was termed the **French disease** or even the **French gout**, the **Neapolitan disease**, and subsequently the **Spanish disease** (in the Netherlands), the **Polish disease** (in Russia), the **Chinese disease** (in Japan), and the **Canton disease** (in China), and even the **Christian disease** (in Turkey). Syphilis, with a rash being a prominent feature of the second stage of the disease, was also called the "**great pox**" to distinguish it from smallpox. A unifying name for the affliction was clearly needed.

The love poem *Metamorphoses*, completed by Ovid in 8 CE, tells of Sipylus, sometimes spelled Siphylus, son of Niobe, who was herself daughter of Tantalus, ruler of the city of Tantalus, near Mount Sipylus in Asia Minor.

A millennium and a half later, in 1530, a Veronese physician, Girolamo Fracastoro, wrote a poem titled *Syphilis sive morbus Gallicus*, which means "Syphilis, the French Disease" (Fig. 2.10). The poem tells of Syphilus, a luckless shepherd boy who, because he had offended Apollo, was stricken with a virulent disease that, as a physician as well as an author, Fracastoro describes in clinical detail, hence the origin of the disease name, **syphilis** (Gershon, p. 100).

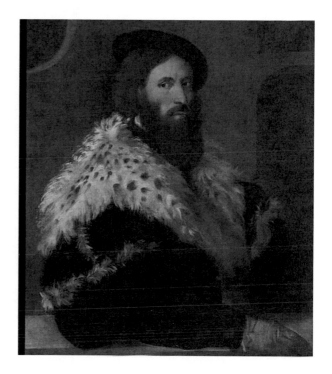

For those readers who are fans of etymologic controversy, Haubrich (p. 218) holds that Syphilus was not a shepherd, but a swineherd, and that lad's name was derived from the Greek word *sypheos*, meaning a "hog sty." Dirckx (p. 58) considers this explanation "implausible," holding that Syphilus was indeed a shepherd.

Ulysses in the Clinic Today

Ulysses, known to the Greeks as Odysseus, was king of Ithaca and a key figure in Homer's *Iliad*. Following the end of the Trojan War, he set out for home. On the journey, his ships are driven off course by storms, and he experiences a host of adventures. He outwits the Cyclops, charms Circe, skirts the land of the Sirens, and wins an archery contest after stringing the bow of Apollo. In short, what began as a routine trip home became a long and perilous journey (Fig. 2.11).

From this classic tale, we derive the eponymous **Ulysses syndrome**. As described by Rang, the initial manifestation is an unexpected abnormality found on laboratory screening or imaging, something that *needs to be checked out* [4]. At this point, the patient is launched on an odyssey of repeat testing, further evaluation, imaging, consultation, second opinions, and occasionally even some sort of invasive procedure. In the end, the patient, if he or she survives the investigative rigors, is relieved to return to his "home" status of good health, knowing by then that all the investigations precipitated by an insignificant incidental finding had been unnecessary, but perhaps relieved to have been declared disease-free.

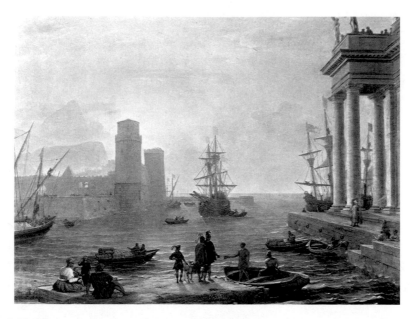

Fig. 2.11 Ulysses departs from the Land of the Phaeacians, the last destination of his 10-year journey before returning home to Ithaca. Public Domain. https://commons.wikimedia.org/wiki/File:Departure_of_Ulysses_from_the_Land_of_the_Pheacians.jpg

Morpheus, the God of Dreams

Another of the ancient gods found in Ovid's *Metamorphoses* is Morpheus, god of dreams or sleep. Although he is, in fact, a winged demon, Morpheus can appear in dreams in human form. The *morph*, meaning "form," in his name refers to the god's ability to shape the dreams appearing to the person sleeping as well as his ability to alter his own body image. The word **morphology**, meaning "the study of the form of things," comes from this source.

Another word we can trace to Morpheus is an alkaloid derived from the opium poppy (Fig. 2.12). In 1816, German apothecary Friedrich Sertürner (1783–1840) isolated a crystalline compound from crude opium; he tested it on dogs with fatal outcomes. He then reduced the dose and tried it himself, one of the many instances of self-experimentation in the long history of medicine. Sertürner experienced both euphoria and pain relief. With the god of sleep in mind, he named the drug **morphine**.

Today the word *morphine* is used as the name of a website blocker, an extension of the website browser Google Chrome. This *morphine* allows the user to block specific websites, essentially putting annoying online content "to sleep."

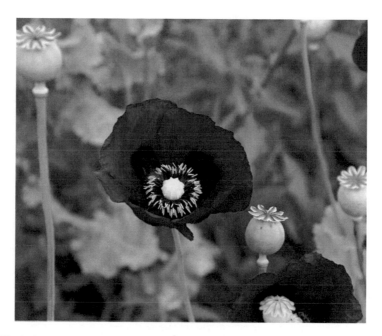

Fig. 2.12 Opium poppy. Photo credit: Tanja Niggendijker, Apeldoorn, The Netherlands. Creative commons. https://commons.wikimedia.org/wiki/File:Papaver_somniferum_flowers.jpg

The Maze and the Inner Ear

A **labyrinth** is either a physical structure of bewildering complexity, such as the legendary labyrinth of Crete, or the complex inner ear structure located in the temporal bone. The word comes from the Greek *labyrinthos*, meaning "maze." And here the story begins.

Greek mythology tells us that legendary craftsman Daedalus built for King Minos of Crete a maze to hold the Minotaur, a fearsome creature with the head of a bull and body of a man. So cleverly did Daedalus construct the maze that he almost failed to escape his own confusing network of paths. We also remember Daedalus because he later constructed wax-and-feather wings for his son, Icarus, who foolishly soared toward the sun, only to have his wings melt, causing him to fall into the ocean and drown, a mythological warning to all of the hazards of hubris.

Crete was not the only site of a **labyrinth**. Herodotus (c. 484–425 BCE) wrote of a complex structure in Egypt that he described as a **labyrinth**. There is evidence that mazes were part of early Indian, Russian, and Native American cultures. A convoluted labyrinthine pattern is found on the floor of French cathedral at Chartres, constructed during the thirteenth century (Fig. 2.13).

With this background, in 1550, Fallopius named the inner ear the **labyrinth** to describe the part of the ear that controls balance and conducts sound from the middle ear to the auditory nerve (Pepper, p. 206).

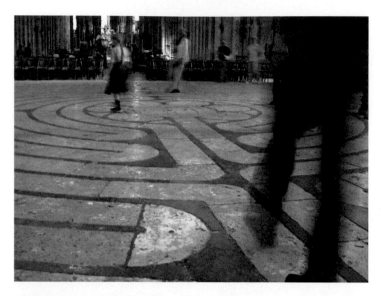

Fig. 2.13 The labyrinth in the Chartres Cathedral. Creative Commons. https://commons.wikimedia.org/wiki/File:Labyrinth_at_Chartres_Cathedral.JPG

The River of Forgetfulness

Five rivers flow through the mythological Greek underworld: Acheron (the river of woe), Cocytus (the river of lamentation), Styx (the river of hate), Phlegethon (the river of fire), and Lethe (the river of forgetfulness). When the dead drank of the River Lethe, they lost all memory of their early life, and only then could they be incarnated.

From the name of this fabled river comes our word **lethargy**, a manifestation of a myriad of diseases.

References

1. Kong R. Apollo 11 disease or acute hemorrhagic conjunctivitis: a pandemic of a new enterovirus infection of the eyes. Am J Epidem. 1975;101:383.
2. Hitti M. Jeremy Piven's high mercury count. WebMD. Available at: http://www.webmd.com/men/news/20081218/jeremy-pivens-high-mercury-count#
3. Nacke P. Die sexuellen perversitaten in der irrenanstalt. Psychiatrische Bladen. 1899;3:122.
4. Rang M. The Ulysses syndrome. CMA Jour. 1972;106:123.

Chapter 3
Descriptive Medical Terms: Activities, Actions, and Appearances

Most medical words lack colorful mythological or even supernatural origins, and many simply arose because an anatomical finding, a disease manifestation, the nature of an organism, or a characteristic of a remedy resembled something familiar to those living at the time. This chapter is about these terms, with some stories of their journeys to the current day. Almost all words described in this chapter come from ancient Greek or Latin roots, although some, such as the word **physician**, have evolved along the way; Chap. 4 tells about words from languages other than the two old classic tongues.

There are countless examples of medical terms that describe things. Here are a few of them:

- The word **ptosis**, a drooping of the eyelid, is the same as the Greek word meaning "a fall" or "falling"; the ptotic eyelid seems to be falling.
- **Cochlea** means "snail" in Latin and earlier came from the Greek word meaning "shape." The cochlea—a spiral-shaped inner ear structure— is shaped like a snail.
- **Clavicle** comes from the Latin word *clavis*, meaning "key." The collarbone shape resembles a key and the bone seems to "lock up" the chest.
- The Latin **biceps** means "two heads," referring to the upper arm muscle with dual origins on the scapula.
- Continuing down the body, we come to the **duodenum**, from Latin *duodeni*, or twelve. This part of the intestine is so named because it is, more or less, 12 fingerbreadths in length.
- **Cuboid**, from a Greek word meaning "cube" combined with a suffix *eidos*, meaning "resemblance," refers to a somewhat square bone in the foot (Fig. 3.1).
- On a different theme, the word **parasite** comes from Greek words *para* ("beside") and *sitos* (food), combined into *parasitos*, meaning someone or something that sponges food from others, just as in microbiology a parasite is an organism that derives nutrients at the host's expense.

© Springer International Publishing AG 2017
R.B. Taylor, *The Amazing Language of Medicine*,
DOI 10.1007/978-3-319-50328-8_3

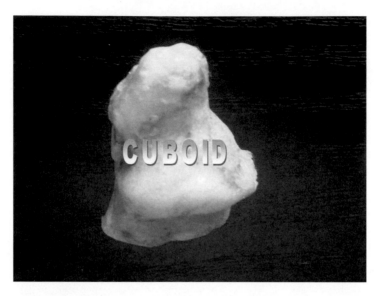

Fig. 3.1 Cuboid bone of the foot. Credit: Anatomist90. Creative Commons. https://commons.wikimedia.org/wiki/File:Cuboid.jpg

Here are more words that describe clinical and scientific entities that remind us of things we see and do in everyday life.

Physician: From Greek to Latin to French to English—To Provider

Our word **physician** has its origins in ancient Greek with the word *physikos*, meaning "natural." In his fictionalized account of the adventures of Hippocrates, *The Torch*, Canadian physician and author Wilder Penfield (1891–1976) quotes his hero, "I am a physician and a teacher of young physicians. Only the Greeks have called their healers by that name. It is a new word and physicians must look to new horizons. *Physis* means nature" [1].

In Latin the word became *physicus*, denoting a physical philosopher. Pepper (p. 119) explains, "in the field of physical philosophy medicine was the zenith." The next iteration was the word *fisicien* in Old French, and then in the early fourteenth century, the English adopted the word *fisitien*, later to become **physician**.

This brings me to the word **doctor**, from the Latin *docere*, meaning "to teach or show." Jamieson tells that the word doctor, as we now know it, was introduced about the year 1200 by French physician Gilles of Corbeil (1140–1224) [2]. There are both bachelor's and master's degrees in medicine, but the highest degree given by the medieval universities in theology, law, or medicine was the doctorate, with the connotation of being a teacher. Today, the best physicians not only diagnose and heal; they also teach their patients.

Then there is a new relatively new term—new, at least in the medical setting—**provider**. The source is the Latin *providere*, meaning "to prepare or supply." The term, intended to foster egalitarianism in health care teamwork, has had the (perhaps) unintended outcome of diminishing the professional primacy of the physician. Nor is use of the term unique to medicine. Aronstein, writing in *American Medical News*, describes provider as "euphemistic nomenclature." He reports, "According to the April 8 (2001) article in the *New York Times Magazine*, both male and female prostitutes in Silicon Valley are referred to as 'providers' by their customers and on their own Web sites" [3].

Plague: Rats, Fleas, Quarantine, and the Black Death

The medical term **plague**, whether used generically or in connection with the disease caused by *Yersinia pestis*, began with the Greek word *plaga*, meaning a "blow." The same word was adopted into Latin to mean a "stroke" or a "wound," and subsequently was used in common parlance to indicate some sort of "pestilence," not far from today's meaning. In the fourteenth century, the era of the Black Death in Europe, *plage* came to describe an "evil scourge" and later a "malignant disease."

The word is also used as a verb: "A stuffy nose has plagued me all winter." And there is a seldom-used adjective, **plaguey**, used to describe something that is vexatious.

The bacterial cause of plague was once named *Pasteurella pestis*, honoring French scientist Louis Pasteur (1822–1895), who helped the world understand the role of microorganisms in disease. I am not sure Pasteur would have been happy to have his name linked to a disease that killed millions throughout history. In 1894, during a plague outbreak in China, Japanese bacteriologist Shibasaburo Kitasato (1853–1931) and Swiss bacteriologist Alexandre Yersin (1863–1943), from the Pasteur Institute, isolated the plague bacillus. The scientific name of the organism was subsequently changed to **Yersinia pestis**, honoring Yersin, but ignoring Kitasato. Both were nominated for a Nobel Prize; neither was awarded the honor.

There were various plagues recorded in the Bible and throughout history, although some of the earlier epidemics may have been caused by something other than *Yersinia pestis*. The most famous outbreak was the so-called **Black Death** that ravaged Europe in the fourteenth century, peaking from 1346 to 1353, perhaps so named for the color of the lesions and the gangrene seen in many victims (Fig. 3.2). The Black Death killed up to 200 million people before running its course, but it gave us two noteworthy things: The first was a book titled *The Decameron*, by Giovanni Boccaccio (1313–1375), a collection of tales told by ten young men and women who fled the plague to shelter in a country villa near Florence, Italy. These three men and seven women spent the long hours of sequestration telling tales, often erotic, of love and life.

Secondly, the Black Death contributed a word to our medical and our everyday vocabulary: **quarantine**. The citizens of Venice soon realized that ships arriving

Fig. 3.2 Acral necrosis of the nose, lips, and fingers and residual ecchymoses over both forearms in a patient recovering from bubonic plague that disseminated to the blood and lungs. Public Domain. https://commons. wikimedia.org/wiki/ File:Acral_necrosis_due_ to_bubonic_plague.jpg

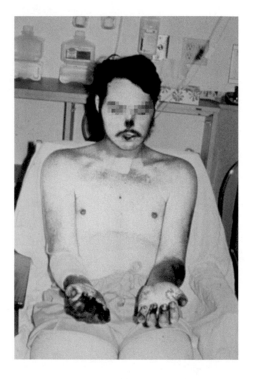

from the Levant often brought infected persons and that the best defense against the disease was isolation. They sealed the port to any vessel suspected of carrying contagion until it had been isolated for 40 days. In Italian, the term for 40 days is *quaranta giorni*, later contracted to *quarantina* (Gershon, p. 82).

Why 40 days? Holt (p. 207) suggests, "There is poetic possibility that the biblical "forty days and forty nights" of flood may have had some occult influence of the choice of that particular number. The prescribed 40 days well exceeds the smallpox incubation period of 7–17 days.

Ascorbic Acid and the Battle Against Scurvy

The action of **ascorbic acid**—the prevention of scurvy—is inherent in the term. The prefix *a-* means "not, without." The root of this term comes from the Medieval Latin word *scorbuticus*, meaning "scurvy." Thus ascorbic acid really means "no scurvy." **Acid** comes from the Latin *acidus*, describing something that tastes sour or sharp, like vinegar, which is, after all, simply diluted acetic acid.

Scurvy is a deficiency disease that occurs owing to the lack of **ascorbic acid**, vitamin C, found in fruits and green vegetables. The disease begins with skin lesions and bleeding gums, followed by lethargy, fever, swollen gums, loss of teeth, neuropathy, and widespread hemorrhage which can cause death. Scurvy was described by Hippocrates (460–377 BCE). Common when persons ate a diet short on green vegetables and fruits, scurvy was a frequent occurrence on long sea voyages, where diets were limited to foods that could be stored for months.

Portuguese explorer Vasco da Gama set out in 1497 to discover a sea route to the East Indies around the southern tip of Africa. Of the 160 men that set out with da Gama, **scurvy** killed approximately 100 during the voyage.

Then in 1519, King Charles I of Spain sent Ferdinand Magellan to circumvent the globe. Of the three ships and 250 sailors that departed Spain, only one ship and eighteen men lived to return home. Antonio Pigafetta (1480–1522), an Italian explorer with Magellan's expedition, wrote of scurvy, "Of all the misfortunes, this was the worst: the gums of some of the men swelled over their upper and lower teeth, so that they could not eat and so died" [4]. Scurvy outbreaks killed about half of the crew, while many others died from conflicts with indigenous peoples.

Scottish physician James Lind (1716–1794), serving as surgeon on the *HMS Salisbury*, suspected that the absence of dietary fruits might be the cause of scurvy. He conducted an experiment on sailors during a long voyage—some received citrus fruits, some did not. Before too long, those sailors who had received fruits in the diet were enlisted to care for those who had not. Lind published his findings, titled *A Treatise on Scurvy*, leading to changes in the diet of English sailors at sea (Fig. 3.3). English sailors subsequently came to be called *Limeys*, even though Lind's experimental group received oranges and lemons—but not limes.

Scurvy was not a problem only for European explorers. In the early nineteenth century, the disease plagued Western American frontier outposts, whose inhabitants ate a diet rich in game meat and poor in vegetables and fruits. The problem of supplying needed antiscorbutic foods continued into the US Civil War.

In the 1920s, Hungarian researcher Albert Szent-Gyorgyi (1893–1986) isolated a substance known as hexuronic acid, subsequently shown to be the chemical key to the prevention of scurvy. Szent-Gyorgyi then created a new name, ascorbic acid, for his chemical discovery, and received the 1937 Nobel Prize in Physiology or Medicine.

Sartorius: the Tailor's Muscle

The **sartorius** muscle takes its name from the Latin word *sartor*, meaning "tailor," and, more specifically, "patcher." This muscle, the longest of the body, helps assist moving a lower extremity to the cross-legged position often assumed by a tailor. Because the muscle is not only long, but thin and ribbon-like, the name may have arisen because of its resemblance to a tailor's measuring tape. Or it may be related to the way tailors measure the inseam when fitting a pant leg. Whatever the pathway from *sartor* to sartorius, the structure is clearly thought of as the "tailor's muscle."

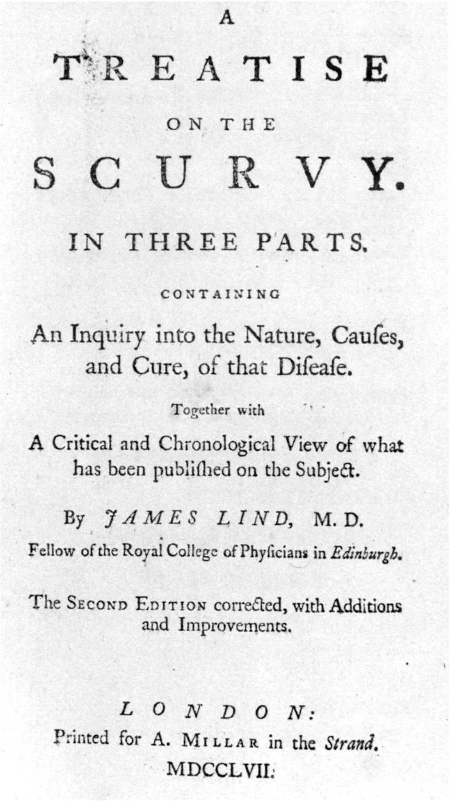

Fig. 3.3 The second
edition of James Lind's
book *A Treatise on Scurvy*.
Source: Wellcome images.
Public Domain. https://
commons.wikimedia.org/
wiki/File:James_Lind,_A_
Treatise_on_the_
Scurvy,_1757_Wellcome_
M0013130.jpg

A

T R E A T I S E

ON THE

S C U R V Y.

IN THREE PARTS.

CONTAINING

An Inquiry into the Nature, Caufes,
and Cure, of that Difeafe.

Together with

A Critical and Chronological View of what
has been publifhed on the Subject.

By *JAMES LIND*, M. D.

Fellow of the Royal College of Phyficians in *Edinburgh*.

The SECOND EDITION corrected, with Additions
and Improvements.

L O N D O N:
Printed for A. MILLAR in the *Strand*.
MDCCLVII.

The Ornithological Origins of the Disease Named Pica

A pathologic tendency to consume items lacking nutritional value is called **pica**. In Latin, the word was the name of the bird commonly known as the magpie (Fig. 3.4). The black-billed magpie consumes a highly diverse diet: seeds, nuts, berries, eggs, rodents, carrion, and even the ticks that infest large animals such as deer or cattle. They seem to ingest almost anything. When food is abundant, magpies hoard uneaten items for later eating. From this, we can see why Swedish zoologist Carl Linnaeus (1707–1778) named the birds *Corvus pica* when first describing them in 1758. *Corvus* means "crow" or "raven" in Latin.

Persons with the disease pica swallow a variety of items, such as chalk, clay, paint, metal, glass, sand, hair, or ice. Children who consume old painted plaster scraped from walls may develop lead poisoning. Bowel obstruction may be caused by hairballs. Many persons with pica have malnutrition and/or anemia. With the diverse variety of ingestants possible in pica patients, it becomes apparent why the disease was named for the bird.

Fig. 3.4 European Magpie *Pica pica* in Gloucestershire, England. Credit: Adrian Pingstone (Arpingstone). Public Domain. https://commons.wikimedia.org/wiki/File:Magpie_arp.jpg

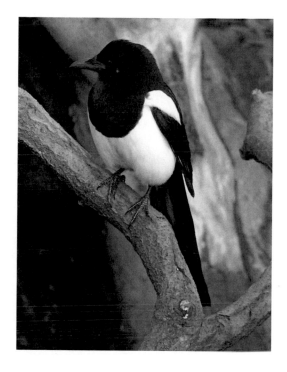

To bring the story up to date, The *Urban Dictionary* describes a magpie as "Someone who hangs at the train station or bus stop or anywhere public all day long, usually asking for a cigarette, spare change, or pocket lint" [5].

Testis, Testimony, and the Swearing on Highly Valued Items

Recently I was called to provide evidence in a trial—to *testify*. Before taking my seat in the witness chair, I was asked to swear on a Bible, with my right hand raised, presumably to Heaven that I would tell "the truth, the whole truth, and nothing but the truth…." The process was not always so.

The source of the words **testis**, **testicle**, and **testify** is the Latin *testis*, meaning "witness." The connection with promising to tell the truth and today's name of an important male body part has biblical origins. In Genesis 24:9 we find, "And the servant put his hand under the thigh of Abraham his master, and sware [sic] to him concerning the matter." But later the picture becomes murky.

There are quaint tales of ancient Greeks, and perhaps later Romans, holding their scrotums while giving evidence at trial. However, the *Online Etymology Dictionary* tells, "Stories that trace the use of the Latin word to some supposed swearing-in ceremony are modern and groundless." Perhaps the more likely link is the assertion that the testicles were witness to/evidence of a man's virility. Whatever the connection, the current custom is to pledge veracity on a holy book, and not on a thigh, reproductive organ, or other body part.

Nausea on the High Seas

In Greek, *naus* meant "ship." Soon *nausia* came to mean "seasickness." Then, about the fifteenth century, the queasy feeling associated with seafaring came to be called **nausea** in Latin. Different than vomiting, nausea is the uneasy feeling that emesis may be eminent.

Nausea, of course, has many causes other than being aboard a ship: gastroenteritis, pregnancy, migraine, food poisoning, bowel obstruction, and medication effects. One online site lists 708 possible causes for the symptom of nausea [6].

Here is an interesting study about the occurrence of nausea: Kennedy et al. studied 10 labyrinthine-defective and 20 normal subjects in the setting of extreme storm conditions during a North Atlantic sea voyage. None of the labyrinthine-defective subjects experienced nausea, while the normal subjects had symptoms of motion sickness, suggesting that the vestibular organs are key factors in the development of seasickness [7].

Perils of Eating Like an Ox

Aristotle wrote of **bulimia** as "ravenous hunger," a word derived from the Greek *bous*, meaning "ox," and *limos*, indicating "hunger." The phrase means to be hungry as an ox. Bulimia, also called **bulimia nervosa**, is an eating disorder in which a person binges (eats like an ox) and then purges the ingested food by vomiting or using laxatives. The disease is most common in young women, those who live in cities, and residents of developed countries.

Ravenous hunger may have been recognized for centuries, but the disease of binge eating followed by purging was first described by British psychiatrist Gerald Russell in 1979, who gave the disorder its name, **bulimia** [8].

There are two noteworthy physical signs that may be seen with bulimia, both related to vomiting. The first is erosion of tooth enamel, damaged by stomach acid during repeated emesis. The second, named the **Russell sign**, is the presence of abrasions and calluses found on the knuckles or back of the hand used to induce vomiting, lesions occurring as the skin is scraped against the patient's maxillary incisors (Fig. 3.5).

The disease described by Russell is an example of how knowing a word's origin can help with spelling. Note the correct spelling: **bulimia**, with two letter "i's." A careless writer might spell the word *bulemia*, like leukemia or anemia, but that would mean "ox blood," not "ox-like hunger."

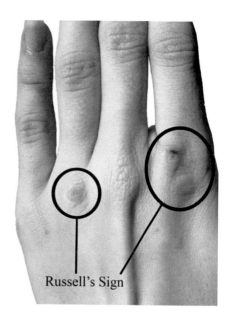

Russell's Sign

Epilepsy, the Not-So-Divine Disease

The word **epilepsy** comes from a Greek root and prefix. The root is *lepsis*, or "seizure"; the prefix is *epi-*, meaning "upon." These combined to give *epilepsis* in Greek and *epilepsia* in Latin. In the sixteenth century, the French word *epilepsie* came into use, and today in English we have **epilepsy**.

Epileptic seizures are found early in history. The son of the god Zeus and the human Alcmene, Hercules is reported to have murdered his children and perhaps (according to which story you read) his wife, Megara, during a fit of epileptic madness. He subsequently atoned for his sins with the legendary 12 Labors. The disease came to have a supernatural aura, and for two millennia, epilepsy was called **Hercules sickness**.

In the fifth century, Hippocrates (460–377 BCE), or perhaps some subsequent acolyte, wrote *On the Sacred Disease*, challenging the notion that epilepsy had a divine origin:

> I am about to discuss the disease called 'sacred.' It is not, in my opinion, any more divine or more sacred than other diseases, but has a natural cause, and its supposed divine origin is due to men's inexperience and to their wonder at its peculiar character [9].

History's most famous epileptic was Russian author Fyodor Dostoevsky (1821–1881), who recorded 102 of his own seizure episodes in his notebook and who included epileptic characters in 4 of his 12 novels. Other reputed epileptics include Alexander the Great of Macedon, Roman emperor Julius Caesar, French emperor Napoleon Bonaparte, US president Theodore Roosevelt, and American author Edgar Allan Poe.

A physician specializing in epilepsy is called an **epileptologist**, a term introduced in 1904 by American neurologist William P. Spratling (1863–1915), thereby becoming the world's first practitioner of this medical specialty.

Islets, Diabetes, and Insulin

In 1869, German anatomist Paul Langerhans (1847–1888) discovered that the pancreas gland was not homogeneous, but contained small areas of tissue that came to be called islets, or small islands. We know these today as the **islets of Langerhans** (Fig. 3.6).

What we now call **diabetes mellitus** was given the Greek name *diabetes* by the second-century physician Aretaeus the Cappadocian, drawing on earlier words meaning to "pass through," to indicate the huge volumes of urine characteristic of uncontrolled disease. The descriptor mellitus is the Latin word for "sweet, honey." Until 1922, what we now call type 1 diabetes was usually a death sentence. The path from the discovery of Langerhans' islets to a game-changing injectable hormone to treat this disease took a half-century.

In 1922, following a series of experiments with dogs, and then a successful trial on a 14-year-old human subject named Leonard Thompson, an extract from the pancreas was recognized as capable of controlling blood glucose levels. The now-famous codiscoverers of this miraculous compound were Nobel laureate Frederick Banting (1891–1941) and his assistant Charles Best (1899–1978). The hormone they isolated and tested successfully was not named by Banting and Best, however, because it had been named prior to its actual discovery. In 1910, English physiologist Sir Edward Albert Sharpey-Shafer (1850–1935) had theorized that the deficiency of a single substance in the pancreas was responsible for diabetes. Postulating that the hypothetical substance originated in the "little islands" of Langerhans, he named it **insulin**, from the Latin *insula*, meaning "island."

The Emperor and the Horse

Claudication, referring to a halting gait or limp, comes from the Latin *claudicare*, meaning "to limp." We use the term most often in the sense of **intermittent claudication**, a limp caused by exercise-induced pain that is soon relieved by rest, classically caused by arterial insufficiency of the leg. According to Caelius Aurelianus, the phenomenon was known to Greek physician Erasistratus (304–250 BCE), sometimes considered the father of physiology, who described it as paradoxical.

Erasistratus terms *paradoxos* (strange, paradoxical) a type of paralysis in which a person walking along must suddenly stop and cannot go on, but after a while can walk again [10].

The name of Roman Emperor Claudius (11 BCE–54 AD) was related to the presence of a severe limp, which might have been due to cerebral palsy or Tourette syndrome (Fig. 3.7).

Fig. 3.6 Human pancreatic islets, visualized using double immunostaining. Colors: red = glucagon antibody, blue = insulin antibody. Creative Commons. https://commons.wikimedia.org/wiki/File:Human_pancreatic_islet.jpg

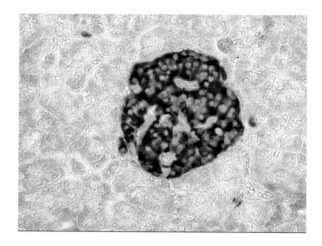

The link to arterial insufficiency was made in 1831 by French veterinarian Jean-François Bouley after observing the curious actions of a horse pulling a cab in Paris. The animal would trot, then collapse. After a short time, the animal would resume its pace and subsequently drop to the ground again. Bouley eventually performed an autopsy on the horse, during which he found a femoral artery obstruction [11].

A few years later, English surgeon and medical writer Sir Benjamin Collins Brodie (1783–1862) brought the term **claudication** to human medicine. We remember Brodie, not for his introduction of a medical word we use today, but for the Brodie abscess, a type of subacute osteomyelitis.

Sydenham, Huntington, and the Chorines

Our word **chorea**, from *khoreia*, a Greek word that means "dance," has been used to name several diseases that manifest uncontrolled, often **athetoid**, movements. The term athetoid, from *athetosis*, means "not fixed, without position or place," and comes from the Greek *athetos* [Online Etymology Dictionary]. There are several diseases with the name **chorea**.

Sydenham chorea—along with polyarthritis, carditis, subcutaneous nodules, and erythema marginatum—is one of the five major manifestations of acute rheumatic fever. This disorder, historically also called **St. Vitus dance** or **chorea minor**, is characterized by uncoordinated movements of the extremities. The eponymous title references British physician Thomas Sydenham (1624–1689), author of *Observationes Medicae*, a reference book used by physicians for two centuries. Saint Vitus is the patron saint of dancers, young persons, and dogs, which seems to me to be an odd portfolio.

Huntington chorea, now called **Huntington disease**, combines choreiform movements with psychiatric and cognitive symptoms. Caused by an autosomal dominant mutation, manifestations generally are first seen during middle age. The disease is named for American physician George Huntington (1850–1916), who described the

Fig. 3.7 Bronze head of
the Emperor Claudius,
found at the River Alde at
Rendham, near
Saxmundham, Suffolk;
British Museum. Credit:
Carole Raddato. Creative
Commons. https://
commons.wikimedia.org/
wiki/File:Bronze_head_of_
the_Emperor_Claudius,_
found_at_the_River_Alde_
at_Rendham,_near_
Saxmundham,_Suffolk,_
British_Museum_
(16250274110).jpg

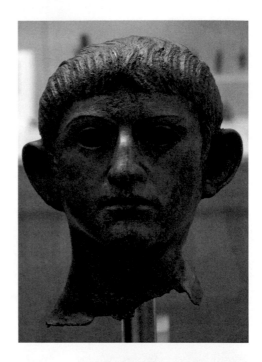

THE

MEDICAL AND SURGICAL REPORTER.

No. 789.]   PHILADELPHIA, APRIL 13, 1872.   [Vol. XXVI.—No. 15.

ORIGINAL DEPARTMENT.

Communications.

ON CHOREA.

By George Huntington, M. D.,
Of Pomeroy, Ohio.

Essay read before the Meigs and Mason Academy of Medicine at Middleport, Ohio, February 15, 1872

Chorea is essentially a disease of the nervous system. The name "chorea" is given to the disease on account of the *dancing* propensities of those who are affected by it, and it is a very appropriate designation. The disease, as it is commonly seen, is by no means a dangerous or serious affection, however distressing it may be to the one suffering from it, or to his friends. Its most marked and char-

The upper extremities may be the first affected, or both simultaneously. All the voluntary muscles are liable to be affected, those of the face rarely being exempted.

If the patient attempt to protrude the tongue it is accomplished with a great deal of difficulty and uncertainty. The hands are kept rolling—first the palms upward, and then the backs. The shoulders are shrugged, and the feet and legs kept in perpetual motion; the toes are turned in, and then everted; one foot is thrown across the other, and then suddenly withdrawn, and, in short, every conceivable attitude and expression is assumed, and so varied and irregular are the motions gone through with, that a complete description of

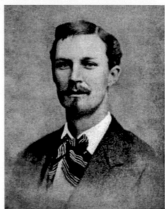

Fig. 3.8 Front page of George Huntington's communication, "On Chorea"; on the right is an 1872 photo of George Huntington. Public Domain. https://commons.wikimedia.org/wiki/File:On_Chorea_with_photo.jpg

disorder in 1872; at this time, Huntington was age 22 and this was his very first medical paper (Fig. 3.8) [12].

We sometimes remember a disease because it has struck a well-known person; for Huntington disease the "famous patient" was folksinger Woody Guthrie, who wrote songs such as "Roll On, Columbia" and "This Land is Your Land."

There is also chorea gravidarum (involuntary movements occurring during pregnancy), choreiform cerebral palsy, and chorea caused by drugs such as anticonvulsants, antipsychotics, and levodopa.

The word roots that are the source of many of our clinical terms are not the exclusive domain of medicine. From the same root, *khoreia*, we have our word chorus. So, the next time you see chorus girls—chorines—dancing on stage, think of the bands of dancers or singers that were a prominent feature of ancient Greek theater.

The Artery of Stupefaction

The **carotid artery** of the neck, carrying blood to the brain, takes its name from the Greek word *karoun*, meaning "to stupefy." Bollett quotes Rufus of Ephesus, who lived in the first century AD, "The ancients called the arteries of the neck *carotides* or *carotikoi* because they believed that when they were pressed hard the animal became sleepy" [13]. Fake healers—mountebanks—in early Greece used to attract crowds and display their powers by squeezing the carotid arteries of a goat until the animal became unconscious, following which there was a prompt return to normal when the pressure was released.

Scottish anatomist John Bell (1763–1820) was skeptical of this story, but in his 1896 book on cerebral circulation, British physiologist Leonard Hill (1866–1952) writes, "Horses, goats, depend entirely upon carotids for their cerebral blood supply, since the vertebrals where they enter the basilar are reduced to mere vascular threads. It has been recorded that occlusion of the carotids only is sufficient to produce spasms and loss of consciousness in these animals. So in spite of Bell's scoffs the mountebanks were in the right" [14]. In humans, the carotids are not, fortunately, the sole blood supply to the brain (Fig. 3.9).

Pudendum, Shame, and Shamelessness

From the Latin word *pudere*, meaning "to be ashamed," we have the anatomical term **pudendum**, and several other words, as well. **Pudendum**, or **pudenda**, for one's "private parts," refers especially to the female genitalia: the mons veneris, the labia majora and minora, and the vaginal orifice. One was supposed to keep these body parts unmentionably modest and certainly not display them shamefully.

From this same root, we have the adjective **pudendal**, referring to the area of the external genitalia, and most often used in regard to the **pudendal block**, an anesthetic injection technique used for vaginal deliveries and local surgery of the vaginal and perineum.

The Roman pantheon included Pudicitia, a goddess who personified the modest virtues of idealized womanhood. She was worshiped at two shrines in Rome,

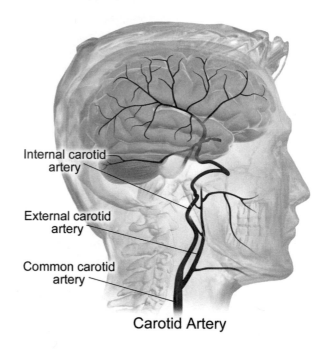

Fig. 3.9 Arterial circulation to the brain. Blausen.com staff. "Blausen gallery 2014." Wikiversity Journal of Medicine. DOI:10.15347/wjm/2014.010. ISSN 20018762. Creative Commons. https://commons.wikimedia.org/wiki/File:Blausen_0170_CarotidArteries.png

Internal carotid artery

External carotid artery

Common carotid artery

Carotid Artery

although both eventually fell into disuse. Although the word is seldom used today, one who is **pudent** is "humble and lacking in ostentation."

On the other side of the coin is **impudent**, meaning "lacking in shame." Although this word is commonly used, I wonder if mothers criticizing their adolescents for being "impudent" recognize the genital history of the word.

The White Plague, Euphemisms, and Poets

Having been found in Egyptian mummies dating to the year 4000 BCE, **tuberculosis** is among our oldest confirmed diseases. In fact, tuberculosis is presumed to have caused the spinal collapse found in a Neolithic skeleton discovered near Heidelberg, Germany. Thus it seems ironic that this enduring and lethal disease takes its name from the humble Latin *tuber*, meaning "lump" or "bump," and shares an etymology with the our word **tuber**, used to describe vegetables such as potatoes. The **tubercles** (literally, little tubers) were, of course, lesions found in the lungs and sometimes in the neck (called scrofula) and spine (Pott disease) (Fig. 3.10).

There has long been a fearful aura surrounding tuberculosis. In the book *Armance*, by Stendhal (a.k.a. Marie-Henri Beyle), we find the mother of a son with the disease who will not utter the word "tuberculosis" for fear of exacerbating his condition [15]. This dread of the disease designation has prompted a number of alternative names, some of which are almost more fearful than the medical word: *consumption* and *white plague* are among them; *phthisis*, *TB*, and *chronic bronchitis*

Fig. 3.10 Scrofula of the neck. From: Bramwell, Byrom Edinburgh, Constable, 1893 Atlas of Clinical Medicine. Source: National Library of Medicine, National Institutes of Health, USA. Public Domain. https://commons. wikimedia.org/wiki/ File:Scrofula.jpeg

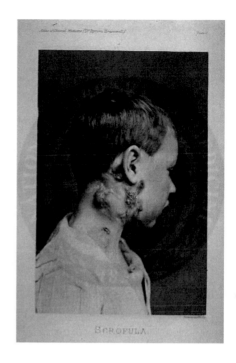

are perhaps more neutral. Other terms related to the disease are clearly euphemisms: calling a sufferer a *lunger* or a *health seeker*, referring to *raising* rather than spitting or *spilling rubies* when one experienced a lung hemorrhage, or being in a *rest ranch* rather than a sanitarium when seeking a cure (Rawson, p. 277).

On the other hand, tuberculosis enhanced the mysticism of many nineteenth-century writers and poets. French writer Alexandre Dumas (1802–1870) wrote, "It was the fashion to suffer from the lungs; everybody was consumptive, poets especially; it was good form to spit blood after each emotion that was at all sensational, and to die before the age of thirty." English poet Lord Byron (1788–1824) once told a friend: "I should like to die of consumption." Why? "Because the ladies would all say: 'Look at that poor Byron, how interesting he looks in dying!'" English poet John Keats (1795–1821) died of tuberculosis at age 26.

Today the ever-resilient tuberculosis is among the leading causes of infection-related deaths worldwide. The World Health Organization estimates that there were almost 10 million new cases in 2014, with 1.5 million deaths.

The Little Mouse of Strength

The descriptive word **muscle** comes from the Latin *musculus*, meaning "little mouse." In Greek, *mys* means both "muscle" and "mouse." It is not hard to envision how an ancient healer might have likened a muscle, especially the body of the biceps muscle, to a "little mouse" under the skin.

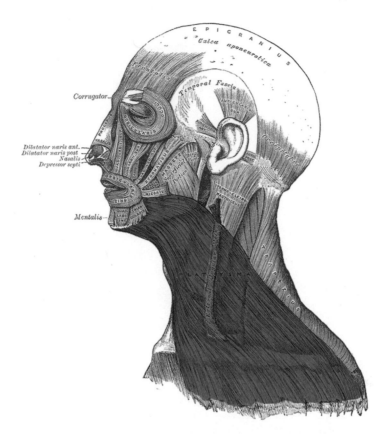

Fig. 3.11 Platysma muscle Source: Gray378.png. Modified by Uwe Gille. Public Domain. https:// commons.wikimedia.org/wiki/File:Platysma.png

There are approximately 640 skeletal muscles in the human body, together comprising some 35–40 % of our body weight. Muscle names have been derived from a number of characteristics of the muscle itself: its shape, for example, the **deltoid muscle** and the **trapezius muscle**; its attachments, the **sternocleidomastoid muscle**; its location, the **frontalis muscle**; and its role, the **flexor carpi ulnaris muscle**.

The name of the **platysma muscle** comes from the Greek *platys*, meaning "flat or broad," a good description of the contractile fibrous bundle in the neck (Fig 3.11). Greek philosopher Plato was named Aristocles at birth, but was later called Plato because of his flat, broad forehead; his breadth of knowledge may also have played a role (Gershon, p. 111).

The Paintbrush that Changed History

Our drug name **penicillin** comes from the Latin *penicillus*, meaning "paintbrush," an apt description of the shape of the fungus *Penicillium notatum*, now called *Penicillium chrysogenum*. Here is the backstory of the name of the antibiotic.

We associate penicillin with Sir Alexander Fleming (1881–1955), who quite accidentally discovered in 1928 that the presence of a mold on his culture plate inhibited the growth of bacteria. Eventually, penicillin became the first bactericidal antibiotic, the first truly effective treatment for syphilis, and a major advantage to the Allies of World War II. In 1944, Fleming was knighted by King George VI of the United Kingdom.

German naturalist Johann Heinrich Friedrich Link (1767–1851) first described the fungal genus *Penicillium* in 1809 [16]. Fleming, indeed, coined the word penicillin. But he simply adapted the earlier term introduced by Link.

Damn the Sphenoid

The **sphenoid** is a prominent bone at the base of the skull, below the frontal lobe of the brain; it is irregular in shape, has two prominent wings, and houses two air-filled sinuses. The bone is more or less wedge-shaped, and takes its name from the Greek *sphen*, meaning "wedge" (Fig. 3.12). This descriptive medical term would not be of much etymologic interest had it not been a favorite topic of a famous medical educator.

"Gentlemen: This is the sphenoid bone. Damn the sphenoid bone." This invective was the first salvo in the annual lecture on the sphenoid to freshmen medical students at Harvard, given by Oliver Wendell Holmes, MD (1809–1894), Parkman Professor of Anatomy from 1847 to 1882, in their course on osteology. Why such harsh words about a small bone?

Writing in 1930, Roddis explained:

> Every physician and student of medicine will know the reason for such profanity in reference to the sphenoid, for with the exception of the temporal bone it is the greatest stumbling block to the medical student in his whole course in osteology. *Cunningham's Anatomy* gives 60 separate facts it is necessary to learn about this small keystone of the skull. There are 64 descriptive facts given about the temporal bone and it is largely a matter of individual taste, or rather distaste, as to which constitutes the worst obstacle to the student [17].

Horses and Sea Monsters

In the medial temporal lobe of the brain, we find the **hippocampus**, concerned with memory and spatial navigation. The word comes from Greek *hippos*, meaning "horse," and *kampos*, or "sea monster," because the structure's shape resembles a seahorse. Pepper (p. 46) tells that this part of the brain was first described by Italian anatomist Costanzo Varolio (1543–1575).

From the same root, we have the medical term **hippus**, an abnormal exaggeration of the rhythmic contraction and dilation of the pupil, which may be benign or might indicate the presence of systemic disease or toxicity. The rhythmic contractions might suggest the movement of a galloping horse. But the etymology becomes a little clearer when we consider that the term **hippus** was formerly applied to nystagmus, which seems a little closer to the experience of horseback riding.

Fig. 3.12 The sphenoid bone. Source: Anatomography. Creative Commons. https:// commons.wikimedia.org/ wiki/File:Sphenoid_ bone_-_close-up_-_ superior_view.png

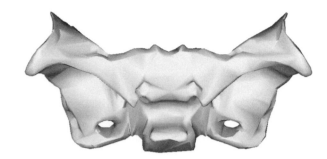

Diphtheria and the Skin of the Goat

In Greek mythology, Amalthea was the she-goat who suckled the infant god Jupiter in a cave in Crete. Later, Jupiter recorded the fate of humankind, writing on the *diphthera* of Amalthea. The Greek word *diphthera* means "skin" or "hide," and when it came time to name an infectious, febrile disease characterized by a pseudo-membrane that looked like a skin in the throat, a logical choice was **diphtheria**.

In literature, **diphtheria** plays a key role in the 1938 short story *The Use of Force* by physician and poet William Carlos Williams (1883–1963). Written in the first person, the story tells of a physician's encounter with a febrile girl who refuses to open her mouth to be examined and who claws at the eyes of the healer trying to help her. The story explores the doctor's love/hate relationship with the child (and her parents) and his feelings about himself as he physically overcomes her resistance, visualizing both tonsils covered with the pseudomembrane of diphtheria [18].

Anal Varicosities and the Ring of Fire

Fundamentally, **hemorrhoids** are varicose veins, and, as such, they can bleed, which explains the word derivation from Greek *haima*, meaning "blood," and *rheo*, signifying "flow," with the connotation of bleeding. In addition to bleeding, hemorrhoids can itch, burn, or hurt. There may be swelling or even thrombosis. Hemorrhoids can be a real pain.

In the Middle Ages, hemorrhoids were known as **Saint Fiacre's curse**, so-called because of the affliction the future saint developed while tilling the soil in the sixth century. Paris taxi drivers regard him as their patron saint. He is also considered the patron saint of gardeners, those with sexually transmitted diseases, and, appropriately, hemorrhoid sufferers (Fig. 3.13).

In 2004, the family of singers June Carter Cash (1929–2003) and Johnny Cash (1932–2003) was approached by a hemorrhoid cream manufacturer. Would the heirs to the rights to Cash's music allow them to use the song "Ring of Fire" in a hemorrhoid remedy commercial? The family was amused, but politely declined.

Fig. 3.13 Saint Fiacre, patron saint of gardeners, hemorrhoid suffers, and others. Mural in Malaga. Public Domain. https://commons.wikimedia.org/wiki/File:Saint_Fiacre_mural,_Seville.jpg

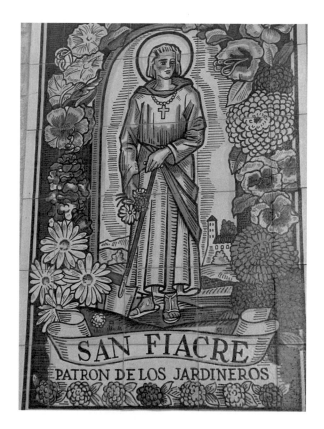

About the Glove of the Fox

The name of the cardiac glycoside **digitalis** comes from the Latin *digitus*, meaning "finger." In 1775, English botanist and physician William Withering (1741–1799) heard of a local Shropshire plant-based cure for dropsy, tested it, and subsequently used it to treat heart failure. The name of the plant was **foxglove**, and Withering published his findings in 1785 as *Account of the Foxglove*.

The origin of the word foxglove is, however, the subject of controversy. Yes, the flowers of the plant *Digitalis purpurea* resemble a glove for a fingertip (Fig. 3.14), but what about the "fox." There are several theories: In the sixteenth century, German botanist Leonhard Fuchs (1501–1566) dubbed the plant "digitalis," harking to the German word *Fingerhut*, meaning "finger hat" or "thimble." But, notice that *Fuchs* in German translates to "fox." Could the name be an eponym for Herr Fuchs? Then there is the suggestion that foxglove is traced to "folk's glove," a theory popularized by Henry Fox Talbot in his 1847 book *English Etymologies*; note the "Fox" in his name, also. Then there is Haubrich (p. 62) telling us that the word foxglove "was so called as early as the eleventh century," predating Withering, Fuchs, and Talbot by several centuries.

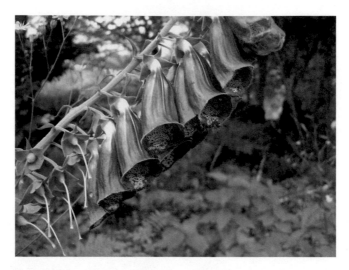

Fig. 3.14 Digitalis purpurea. Credit: Isidre Blanc. Creative Commons. https://commons.wikime-dia.org/wiki/File:DIGITALIS_PURPUREA_-_ARTIGA_LIN_-_IB-071_(Digital).JPG

The Tale of the Tailbone

The final three to five rudimentary vertebrae of the spinal column—generally fused, sometimes separate—comprise the **coccyx**, formally known as *os coccyges*, or the tailbone. A vestige of the tail found in other mammals, the **coccyx** serves as the site of attachment for several muscles and ligaments. The name of the bone is from the Greek *kokkux*, "the cuckoo bird." The bone seems to resemble a cuckoo's bill in shape, as told in the writings of the Greek physician Herophilus (335–280 BCE). In the sixteenth century, Italian anatomist Andreas Vesalius (1514–1564) used the term *os cuculi*, meaning "cuckoo bone" in Latin.

Trauma to the coccyx can cause a painful condition called **coccydynia**, a term derived from *coccyx* plus *–dynia*, from the Greek *odyne*, meaning "pain."

Shutting the Window of Vision

According to the US National Institutes of Health, **cataracts** are the leading cause of visual impairment in the world. A cataract is a cloudiness of the lens causing dim vision, faded colors, and glare. By age 80, more than half of all Americans will have cataracts or have had cataract surgery.

The word cataract comes from the Greek *kataraktes*, a "waterfall," in turn derived from *kata*, "down," and *arassein*, "to dash." A cataract can be said to shut down the window of vision. Or perhaps the person with cataracts sees things as if looking through a waterfall.

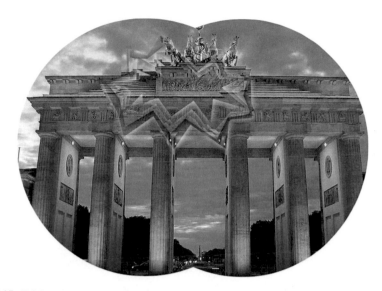

Fig. 3.15 Teichopsia. Note the "fortification" pattern in the visual field. Author: S. Jähnichen. Source: Brandenburger_Tor_Blaue_Stunde.jpg. Creative Commons. https://commons.wikimedia. org/wiki/File:Fortifikation_(Migräne).jpg

The word cataract has also retained its meaning of "a large waterfall." Think of Angel Falls in South America, Victoria Falls in Africa, and Niagara Falls in North America—all are technically classified as cataracts.

A Vision of a Fort

The image of zigzag lines in the visual fields is called **teichopsia**, coming from the Greek *teikhos*, or "wall," and *opsis*, meaning "sight." Also sometimes called a **fortification pattern**, the phenomenon takes its name from the resemblance of the pattern to the battlements of a castle or a walled medieval town as seen from above (Fig. 3.15).

Teichopsia is most often seen as part of the migraine aura, the visual and perhaps other events that precede the onset of head pain. Also, a surprisingly large number of persons have **acephalgic migraine**—migraine without headache—that is manifested solely by a few minutes of visual phenomena such as **teichopsia**, only to note that the visual symptom subsides without subsequent head pain or other problems.

The word **migraine** itself comes originally from the Greek *hemikrania*, the combination of the prefix *hemi-*, "half," and *kranion*, or "skull," consistent with migraine headaches classically being one-sided. Although we do not know if American statesman and president Thomas Jefferson (1743–1826) had **teichopsia** as part of an aura, we do know from his writings that he had severe, recurring headaches that were probably migraines. They often occurred at the time of important historical events, including when Jefferson was drafting the Declaration of Independence.

Ears, Goats, and Tragic Flaws

The small protrusion of the external ear situated anterior to the concha is the **tragus**. Its function is to direct sound waves coming from behind into the auditory canal; these sound waves arrive a little later than those coming from the front, helping one to discern the source of sounds heard. The word comes from Greek *tragos*, meaning a "he-goat." Note the gender specificity. He-goats, like "he-men," have beards. Because the prominence on the external ear is pointed, like a chin, and often has hairs, especially in older men, it seemed to resemble a goatee, hence the name **tragus**, from "goat."

The writings of Roman poet Ovid (43 BCE–17 CE), specifically *The Fasti*, *Tristia*, *Pontic Epistles*, *Ibis*, and *Halieuticon*, mention a fish called the *tragus*, presumably because of a bearded, goat-like facies.

From the same root, we have our word **tragedy**, a tale related formally, with an unhappy ending classically related to the hero's character flaw, or "tragic flaw," leading to his or her downfall. The goat/*tragos* connection comes from the Greek plays in which some performers dressed in goatskins as satyrs—half man and half goat.

The Body's Holy Bone

Of all 206 bones in the human body, only one is considered holy—the **sacrum** (Fig. 3.16). The sacrum, located below the lumbar vertebrae and superior to the coccyx, was named *hieron osteon*, "holy bone," by the Greeks. The Romans called it the *os sacrum*, the "sacred bone." Why was it considered sacred? Several different explanations are offered.

In Greek, the word *hieron* had several meanings: One was "sacred," but another was "temple." In the sense that the female organs of procreation were nestled in the *hieron osteon*, the bone was sacred, a sort of a holy temple.

Gershen (p. 6) tells that the sacrum, owing to its large size, is the last bone to crumble in a decomposing body and hence would serve as the nidus around which a new body would be formed in the afterlife.

In an alternative theory, Dirckx (p. 49) holds that the bone derives its name from "the custom of offering this part of a sacrificial animal on the altar." Thus the gods would be pleased for the gift of this special bone. Another possibility is that the sacrum was used to hold sacrificed materials in ancient sacred rites and hence took on a "holy" aura of its own.

Whatever the true etymological path taken, the word **sacrum** is firmly imbedded in our medical language.

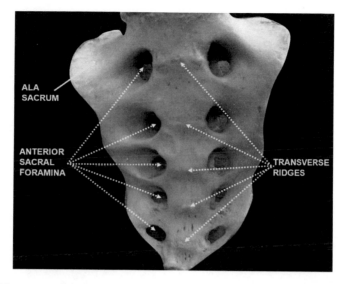

Fig. 3.16 The sacrum. Credit Anatomist90. Creative Commons. https://commons.wikimedia.org/wiki/File:Slide2CORO.JPG

Beware of the Mad Dog

In Latin, the word **rabies** means "mad", it comes from the infinitive *rabere*, meaning "to be mad or to rage." The viral disease **rabies**, historically spread by "mad" dogs and other infected animals, affects chiefly the nervous system. The disease is carried in saliva and typically occurs when one infected animal bites another or perhaps a human. Symptoms include confusion, violent movements, and apparent rage. The victim appears "mad." Glottal spasm and involuntary contraction of the muscles of swallowing when attempting to drink can produce the sometimes-described "foaming at the mouth" feared in mad dogs, giving rise to the term **hydrophobia**. If untreated, the disease is often fatal (Fig. 3.17).

Rabies has been with us for a long time. Pepper (p. 133) tells that it was known to Hippocrates (460–377 BCE) and described by Celsus (25 BCE–50 CE). Folk legend and the 1897 novel *Dracula* by Bram Stoker depict the werewolf as a man by day who transforms to a ferocious wolf at the time of a full moon. Ciardi (p. 410) suggests that the werewolf is "probably a semi-mythological figure personifying rabies."

The first **rabies vaccine** was developed in 1885 and was tested by Louis Pasteur (1822–1895) on 9-year-old Joseph Meister, who had been badly bitten by a rabid dog. The boy survived, and the connection between the young man and Pasteur endured; the rabies survivor spent his career as gatekeeper at the Pasteur Institute in Paris. At age 64, Meister took his own life shortly after the Nazis invaded Paris.

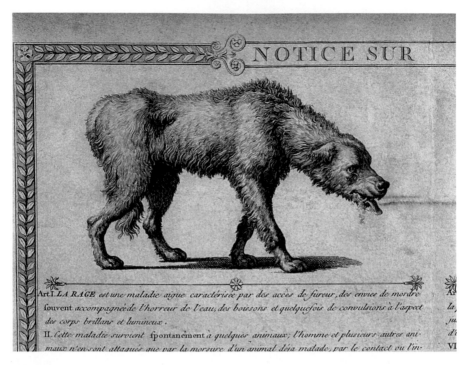

Fig. 3.17 A dog with rabies. Source: Wellcome Trust. Creative Commons. https://commons.wiki-media.org/wiki/File:A_dog_with_rabies_and_a_detail_of_its_skull._Line_engraving_Wellcome_V0010532.jpg

Sewing and Seams

The word **suture**, coming from the Latin *sutura*, "seam," has several related meanings. It can mean a joint between two bones, such as in the skull; a series of stitches joining two edges of an incision or laceration; or the act of placing the stitches.

The use of sutures in the skin is not new. Claudius Galen (129–200) used material made from animal intestines, or "gut," as sutures, and in the tenth century, Persian physician Muhammad ibn Zakariya al-Razi, better known as Rhazes, described the use of harp strings as sutures (Pepper, p. 150).

So-called catgut sutures have the advantage of being absorbable and thus are used when suture material cannot be removed. The "catgut" suture material was made from the fibrous layer of the small intestines of barnyard animals or from beef tendons. The guts of cats were probably never used, and the "cat" in catgut seems to have come from the word *kit*, used in the sixteenth century to describe a "small fiddle," itself derived from Greek *kithara*, meaning "guitar." Today we are much more likely to close wounds with synthetic suture material instead of processed animal parts.

References

1. Penfield W. The torch. Boston. Little, Brown; 1960, p. 192.
2. Jamieson HC. Catechism in medical history. Can Med Assoc J. 1942;47:373.
3. Aronstein WS. Oldest profession prefers "provider." Amer Med News. 2001: May 21, p. 38.
4. Pagafetta A. Journal of Magellan's Voyage. The original text of the Ambrosian manuscript. Translated by James Alexander Robertson, Cleveland: The Arthur H. Clark Company; 1906.
5. Urban Dictionary. Definition of Magpie. http://www.urbandictionary.com/define.php?term=Magpie
6. Differential diagnosis: Nausea. Available at: http://en.diagnosispro.com/differential_diagnosis-for/poisoning-specific-agent-nausea/37707-154-100.html
7. Kennedy RS, Graybiel A, McDonough RC, Beckwith FD. Symptomatology under storm conditions in the North Atlantic in control subjects and in persons with bilateral labyrinthine defects. Acta Otolaryngol. 1968;66(6):533–40.
8. Russell G. Bulimia nervosa: An ominous variant of anorexia nervosa. Psychological Med. 1979;9:429.
9. Hippocrates. On the sacred disease. Translated by Francis Adams. Available at: https://en.wikisource.org/wiki/On_the_Sacred_Disease
10. Aurelianus C. On acute and chronic diseases. Edited and translated by Drabkin IE. Chicago: Univ of Chicago Press; 1950, p. 575.
11. Sugar O. Jean-François Bouley (Bouley jeune): pioneer investigator in intermittent claudication. Spine. 1994;19:346.
12. Huntington G. On chorea. Medical and Surgical Reporter of Philadelphia. 1872;26:317.
13. Bollett AJ. Lessons in medical history. Resident and Staff Phys. 1999;45(9):60.
14. Hill L. The physiology and pathology of the cerebral circulation: an experimental research. London: Churchill. 1896; p. 119.
15. Stendahl. Armance. New York: CreateSpace Independent Publishing Platform; 2015.
16. Link JHF. Observationes in ordines plantarum naturales. Dissertatio I. Magazin der Gesellschaft Naturforschenden Freunde. (in Latin). Berlin. 1809;3:3.
17. Roddis LH. Medicine and the muse: Oliver Wendell Holmes, MD. Ann Int Med. 1930;3:717.
18. Williams WC. The use of force. In: Life along the Passaic River. New York: New Directions; 1938.

Chapter 4
Medical Words from Various Languages

Some of our most colorful and intriguing clinical terms have arisen from languages of diverse countries around the globe. We use words from German, such as **mittelschmerz**, literally "pain in the middle," to describe the pain of ovulation that occurs in the middle of the menstrual cycle. Our word **dengue**, the name of a mosquito-borne febrile illness, comes from West Indian Spanish, and the word probably traveled there with slaves brought from Africa. **Yaws**, an infectious disease with berry-like lesions, probably also comes from an African word meaning "berry." There are a number of English terms used clinically. Some, such as **head, gut,** and **knee,** are from Old English; these are good, time-tested, one-syllable words. More recent clinical terms arising from modern English are often descriptive: **Chinese restaurant syndrome, tennis elbow,** and **runner's knee**.

With the disclaimer that some etymologic purists may espouse antecedents in ancient languages that seem to predate my modern language attributions, here are some words from five continents and Oceania and exotic entries in our medical dictionary that did not come directly from ancient Greek or Latin.

Rumors, Noises, and Hums

Our word **bruit** comes to medicine from Old French, and we have retained the French pronunciation. There is no "it" in bruit. An early, now archaic, definition of the word was "rumor" or "hearsay." William Shakespeare (1564–1616) writes in *Henry VI, Part III*:

> Brother, we will proclaim you out of hand:
> The bruit thereof will bring you many friends. (Act IV, Scene7)

Later, the term bruit came to mean a noise, especially an abnormal one. It was not long before medicine appropriated the word to denote the sound made by turbulence of the blood in an artery or the heart. When you think about it, it isn't too great

© Springer International Publishing AG 2017
R.B. Taylor, *The Amazing Language of Medicine*,
DOI 10.1007/978-3-319-50328-8_4

a leap from the interpersonal turmoil that can attend a rumor to turbulence in the circulatory system.

In 1848, American physician and writer Oliver Wendell Holmes, Sr. (1809–1894), gave us "The Stethoscope Song: a Professional Ballad," in which he mentions several types of bruits known to physicians of his day:

The *bruit de râpe* and the *bruit de scie*
And the *bruit de diable* are all combined;
How happy Bouillaud would be,
If he a case like this could find!

For the record, Jean-Baptiste Bouillaud (1796–1881) was a French physician and researcher who pioneered identifying the roles of various areas of the brain.

I am sad to report that today's would-be physicians seldom learn about the *bruit de scie*, which sounds like a saw, or the *bruit de diable*, the devil's noise. Modern young physicians are hearing "One look is worth a thousand listens" and beginning to question the value of the stethoscope. Will the day come when the study of the bruit becomes an anachronism?

Druggists and Grocers

In Old French, *apotecaire* describes a merchant who compounds and dispenses medications. Here is an instance in which the etymologic stickler might challenge my placing the word in this chapter: The French word comes from Latin *apothecarius*, meaning storekeeper, but lacking the "druggist" connotation. And there is an earlier Greek word *apotheke*, meaning "storehouse." Eventually one who dispensed medications came to be called an **apothecary**.

It was not until 1617 that the Apothecaries' Company of London broke with the Grocers and became true pharmacists dispensing the compounds available in their day (Fig. 4.1). There was competition between physicians and apothecaries, but the latter gained public favor during the Great Plague of London in 1665. At that time, according to Garrison (p. 292), "when the apothecaries made good in public estimation by staying at their posts, while the physicians (even Sydenham) fled for their lives."

Still, by often charging high prices for remedies that had little therapeutic value, the apothecaries were not held in uniformly high regard. In 1796, in his *A Classical Dictionary of the Vulgar Tongue*, English lexicographer Francis Grose (1731–1791) criticized "the assumed gravity and affectation of knowledge generally put on by the gentlemen of this profession, who are commonly as superficial in their learning as they are pedantic in their language."

Today, we seldom speak of the apothecary; the current term is **pharmacist** in American English and **chemist** in British English.

Fig. 4.1 Apothecaries hall in London. Source: R. Sones. Creative Commons. https://commons.wikimedia.org/wiki/File:Apothecaries_Hall_entrance,_Black_Friars_Lane_EC4_-_geograph.org.uk_-_1271897.jpg

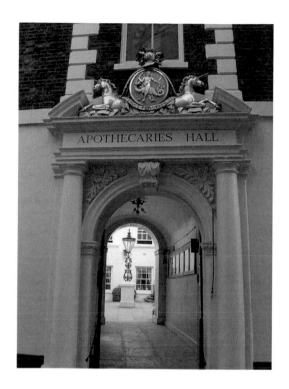

Making a Crackling Sound

Another endangered word we inherited from the French is **rales**. In French, the word is *râle*, from the infinitive *râler*, meaning "to make a rattling sound." In 1816, French physician René Laennec (1781–1826), inventor of the stethoscope, introduced the word into the medical vocabulary to describe what he heard as he examined chests using his monaural invention (Fig. 4.2). In English, we simply adopted the French word, minus the diacritical mark.

One of my 1950s medical school professors described the sound of normal vesicular breathing as like wind rustling through leaves. Rales, abnormal rattling sounds, are often modified with adjectives, such as moist, dry, gurgling, or clicking. Sibilant rales are a whistling or hissing sound. Fine cracking rales are described as crepitant, from Latin *crepitare*, meaning "to rattle." In his book *Mortal Coils*, published in 1922, English author Aldous Huxley (1894–1963) writes, "The air was fairly crepitating with humour." Coarse rales are sometimes likened to the sound of opening a Velcro fastener.

In his day, probably no one had previously heard rales more clearly than did Laennec following his 1816 invention of the stethoscope—first devised using a rolled piece of paper to listen to the chest of an overweight young woman, in whom the direct application of his ear to her chest would have been quite unseemly. Later, in a twist of fate, Laennec was one of many of his time to suffer tuberculosis. His

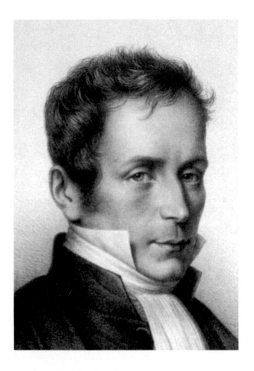

Fig. 4.2 René Laennec (1781–1826), inventor of the stethoscope. Public Domain. https://commons.wikimedia.org/wiki/File:Rene_Laennec.jpg

cousin, French physician Mériadec Laennec (1797–1873), made the diagnosis using Laennec's stethoscope.

But the term rales is in jeopardy. In 1977, despite all the colorful history and clear line of authorism, in what might have been a fit of Francophobia, the American College of Chest Physicians and the American Thoracic Society jettisoned the word rales and installed **crackles** as the preferred term. Somehow this new term lacks the élan of rales. *Dommage, mes amis.*

Hospital

A commonly encountered word that came directly from Old French is **hospital**, then meaning "a place of shelter" or "a lodging" and coming from earlier Latin *hospitalis*. Certainly today, the hospital is a place of housing for the sick. Our word **hospitality** comes from the same root. In 1873, the suffix *–ize* was added to give us **hospitalize**.

There have been lodging places where the sick and wounded came for care since the time of the early Egyptians and Greeks. The latter built *Asclepieia*, temples of healing dedicated to the god Aesculapius; the remains of these structures can be visited today at a number of sites in Greece, including Epidaurus and the Island of Kos.

When the Romans came to conquer Britain, they brought with them the concept of the hospital. Later, in medieval times, hospitals donned a cloak of religiosity and a commitment to serve the poor.

One hospital that has been involved with a medical word is the Pitié-Salpêtrière Hospital in Paris, which began as a gunpowder factory and was eventually converted into a world-class hospital that treated the rich and famous, such as Prince Rainier of Monaco and Diana, Princess of Wales. The Old French word *salpetre* meant "salt of rock," the name used for potassium nitrate, also called **saltpeter**, an ingredient in gunpowder that gave the hospital its name. The chemical's ability to inhibit *C. botulinum* has been important in preserving meat products. There is, however, no known support for the folk legend that **saltpeter** is an anaphrodisiac that causes erectile dysfunction.

What is Done When There is not Enough Care for All

Another word taken directly from French, and one likely to continue in use, is **triage.** The word comes from the French *trier*, meaning to "winnow or cull," and originally referred to the grading of agricultural products. By the eighteenth century, the term was widely used to describe the process of sorting coffee beans into three categories, with the lowest grade, mostly damaged beans, dubbed "triage coffee" (Rawson, p. 287).

In the bloody battlefields of World War I, the French army adopted the term triage to describe sorting the wounded. In his 1976 book *The Face of Battle*, British military historian and author John Keegan (1934–2012) writes that triage "required surgeons, from the press of casualties flowing in during a battle, to send on those who could stand the journey and to choose, from the group remaining, which men were worth subjecting to serious surgery and which must be left to die; the greater the press of casualties, the larger the latter group" (Fig. 4.3).

In today's emergency departments, a key member of the staff is the **triage nurse**. If you have chest pain or active bleeding, you go to the head of the line. Someone with abdominal pain or high fever may come next. The patient with a skin rash or sore throat may be triaged to wait quite a long time.

Sausages, Books, and Botox

American novelist Harlan Coben (born 1962) has said, "A novel is like a sausage. You might like the final taste but you don't want to see how it was made." Similar comparisons have been made with regard to litigation and legislation. The word **botulism** comes from the German *botulismus*, coming into the German language from the Latin *botulus*, meaning "sausage." And there is a story.

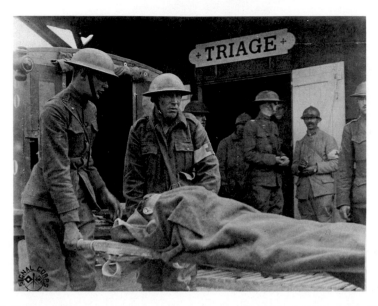

Fig. 4.3 Wounded arriving at a triage station in France, World War I. Author: Otis Historical Archives National Museum of Health and Medicine. Creative Commons. https://commons.wikimedia.org/wiki/File:Wounded_Triage_France_WWI.jpg

The risks of sausage consumption were recognized early in history. In the tenth century, Emperor Leo VI of Byzantium prohibited the manufacture of blood sausages. Following late nineteenth-century outbreaks of "sausage poisoning" in Southern Germany, notably in Württemberg, Germans began to recognize the risks of eating poorly preserved and undercooked pork products.

In 1895, Belgian bacteriologist Émile van Ermengem (1851–1932) isolated the organism that causes botulism from pork products that had poisoned 34 people. He named it *Bacillus botulinus*, but the name was later changed to *Clostridium botulinum*. The genus name *Clostridium* comes from the Greek *kloster*, meaning "spindle"; the organism resembles the spindle used in weaving cloth (Fig. 4.4). Because of the association of the organism with sausage, he named the disease botulism.

Botulinum toxin causes, among other manifestations, muscle weakness and even paralysis. This property of the toxin has been harnessed as botulinum toxin (Botox), used in cosmetic treatments and as therapy for an odd assortment of diseases including migraine headache, strabismus, hyperhidrosis, blepharospasm, bruxism, anal fissure, vaginismus, and obesity.

The Pox, Great and Small

British politician John Montagu, Fourth Earl of Sandwich (1718–1792), once challenged English statesman John Wilkes (1725–1797), "Sir, I do not know whether you will die on the gallows or of the pox." Wilkes is reported to have replied, "That

Fig. 4.4 Photomicrograph of *Clostridium botulinum* bacteria stained with Gentian violet. Centers for Disease Control and Prevention. Public Domain. https://commons. wikimedia.org/wiki/ File:Clostridium_ botulinum.jpg

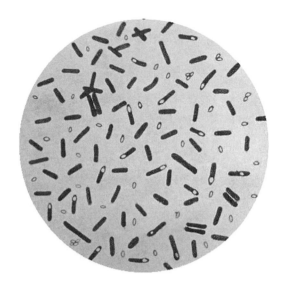

depends, my lord, on whether I embrace your lordship's principles or your mistress."

The word **pock**, plural **pox**, came into English from the Early German *pu (h)*, meaning to "swell up." In English, usage of the word *pocc* was refined to mean some sort of "pustule" or "blister." In the days of Montagu and Wilkes, two types of pox were widespread. The first was **smallpox**, also called the "speckled monster" in the eighteenth century, when the disease killed some 400,000 persons annually and left the survivors scarred and sometimes blind. The disease raged periodically until the advent of vaccination, introduced by English general practitioner Edward Jenner (1749–1823) in 1796 (Fig. 4.5).

The "speckled monster" was called smallpox to distinguish it from the "great pox"—**syphilis**, as described in Chap. 2. Over the years, syphilis was treated with a variety of remedies, with mercury and later arsenicals (Salvarsan) being the most popular. Only with the availability of penicillin in the 1940s did we have a real remedy for the great pox. Yet, in 2014, the Centers for Disease Control and Prevention reported 63,450 new cases of syphilis in the United States, more than the estimated new cases of human immunodeficiency virus infection (HIV) or gonorrhea [1].

Tobacco as Cure and Curse

I hereby declare **tobacco** a medical word because it was introduced to Europe as a cure for gout and other maladies and because we have since learned it to be a cursed cause of lung cancer and other pulmonary and cardiovascular diseases.

Tobacco use in the Americas dates to before 1000 BCE, according to archeological findings in Mexico, and was part of the culture of many Native American tribes.

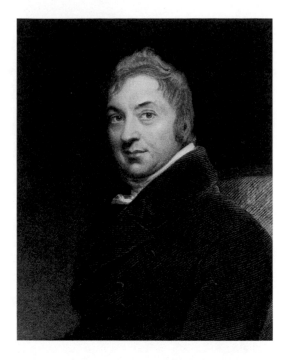

Fig. 4.5 Edward Jenner
(1749–1823). Public
Domain. https://commons.
wikimedia.org/wiki/
Edward_Jenner#/media/
File:Edward_Jenner2.jpg

The plant was unknown in Europe until it was encountered by Christopher Columbus in 1492 and later imported from the New World in the middle of the sixteenth century. Tobacco takes its name from the Spanish *tobaco*, meaning "large tube," referring to the tubular pipe with which the Indians smoked the crushed leaves. The Spanish word may have come from the Taíno language spoken by indigenous persons in the Caribbean islands.

The tobacco plant is *Nicotiana tabacum* and the active ingredient is **nicotine**, both named for Jean Nicot de Villemain, French ambassador in Portugal, who in 1560 championed tobacco use in France, espousing its medicinal value. Queen mother Catherine de Medici began using the product to treat her migraines, and the habit of tobacco use caught on. In 1635, Italian scholar Giambattista della Porta (1535–1615) wrote: "Tobacco allays the cruel tortures of the gout... The leaves cure rotten Sores and Ulcers... doth also presently take away and asswage the pain in the codds" [2].

Tobacco was smoked as prophylaxis during the plague epidemics that followed the plant's introduction into Europe. And according to Jamieson, in the eighteenth century, the smoke was blown into the vagina to treat diseases in this area. Rectal insufflations of **tobacco** smoke were used to treat intestinal diseases. Jamieson describes, "Textbook illustrations show the patient smoking his pipe and by means of a long tube puffing the smoke into his rectum" [3]. It was also used as insect repellant, until replaced by more effective and less harmful chemicals in the 1980s.

As a reward for his popularizing a noxious weed, the French scientific community honored their ambassador by naming the toxic chemical nicotine.

Today we know the truth about tobacco and nicotine. Cigarette smoking is a factor in about one-fifth of all deaths in the United States, and tobacco use is the leading preventable cause of death in this country.

The Flowering Plant That Gave Us Mary Jane

So-called "medical marijuana" is now part of our therapeutic arsenal. The word **marijuana** comes from Mexican Spanish, *marihuana*. Yes, there is a difference between the language of Spain, or "peninsular Spanish," and Mexican Spanish. Sometimes different words are used for the same thing, as in these examples:

Snacks: *Tapas* in Peninsular Spanish, *botanas* in Mexican Spanish
Prawn: *Gamba* in Peninsular Spanish; *camarón* in Mexican Spanish
Pen: *Bolígrafo* in Peninsular Spanish; *pluma* in Mexican Spanish

The *Oxford English Dictionary* suggests that the plant name was derived from the word *mallihuan*, meaning "prisoner" in the Nahuatl language of Mesoamerican indigenous people, but this derivation is disputed. The *Online Etymology Dictionary* tells that in 1918, influenced by the Spanish, marijuana was sometimes called *Maria Juana*. Later aficionados sometimes called it "Mary-John," suggesting aphrodisiac properties (Pepper, p. 103). The echoic term "Mary Jane" is still heard today. In 1938, we saw the first use of the word **pot** as slang for marijuana. In this setting, pot comes from the Mexican Spanish word *potiguaya*, meaning "marijuana leaves."

The drug comes from the flowering herb *Cannabis*, a word derived from the Greek *kannabis*, meaning "hemp." Cannabis, in addition to giving us marijuana, is a source of hemp fiber and oils (Fig. 4.6).

Marijuana has been used for thousands of years, notably in India and Nepal. Today, we not only have medical marijuana—used to treat chronic pain, nausea, and vomiting associated with chemotherapy and anorexia in patients with HIV. We in the United States also have recreational marijuana, legal in four states and the District of Columbia at the time of this writing.

From Brazil to Your Medicine Cabinet, and Then Not

The Portuguese word *igpecaya* was shortened in English to give us **ipecac**, a drug used to induce vomiting, especially following poisoning. The earlier form of the word was *ipecacuanha* in the language of the Tupi people of Brazil, appropriated along with the rest of the culture by the conquering Portuguese. The drug comes from the *Carapichea ipecacuanha* plant that grows in Brazil and several nearby countries.

The Western world first learned of ipecac when mentioned by a Portuguese friar in *Purchas his Pilgrimes*, penned in 1625 by English cleric and travel writer Samuel

Fig. 4.6 Marijuana plant.
Photo by Jorge Barrios.
Public Domain. https://
commons.wikimedia.org/
wiki/File:Marijuana_plant.
jpg

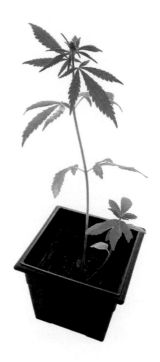

Purchas (1577–1626). Garrison (p. 290) goes on to tell, "About 1680, it began to be extensively prescribed as a secret remedy for dysentery." Later, ipecac was mixed with opium to create **Dover's powder**, used to treat colds and fever. Dover's powder was the brainchild of physician Thomas Dover (1662–1742), the notorious "pirate doctor" who raided towns on the west coast of South America in 1709 (Taylor, 2016, p. 287).

During my early practice years in the 1960s, it was recommended that families keep a small bottle of **ipecac syrup** in the home to use as first aid in case of accidental poisoning. As the father of two small children, I carefully followed this advice, even after one (unnamed adult) family member, in the middle of the night, mistook the **ipecac** bottle for cough syrup, with predictable results. Current guidelines from the American Academy of Pediatrics and other learned organizations now advise against this practice.

More Potent than Marijuana

Marijuana comes from one species of the *Cannabis* plant; **hashish** comes from another. The source of hashish, *Cannabis indica*, was named in 1785 by French naturalist Jean-Baptiste Lamarck (1744–1829), after discovering specimens of the plant in India. *Cannabis sativa*, the source of marijuana, grows tall with ranging branches. In contrast, *Cannabis indica* grows shorter, has broad leaves, and is more adapted to the climates of India, Pakistan, Bangladesh, and Pakistan, where it was cultivated for the production of hashish.

The word hashish comes directly from the Arabic word *hashish*, meaning "powdered hemp" or "hay." In hashish, we find tetrahydrocannabinol (THC) and other cannabinoids, but in concentrations greater than are present in marijuana. In short, hashish is marijuana on steroids. As recently as the 1970s, hashish was sold legally in some Asian countries (Fig. 4.7).

Our word **assassin** has its roots in hashish. About the twelfth century, the Arabs used the word *hashishin*, meaning "rabble," as a derogatory term to refer to their enemies, perhaps suggesting their use of the drug. The word came to describe a secret order of the Middle Eastern Nizari Ismailis, warriors especially trained in killing. Eventually used by the Crusaders, the term evolved into the word assassin, meaning one who is a professional murderer.

Eye Shadow and Demons

Another word that comes from Arabic is **alcohol**. Isn't it curious that the names of some of the world's most popular mind-altering drugs come from languages other than ancient Greek and Latin? The source of alcohol in Arabic is *al-koh'l*, meaning "to paint," with specific reference to a fine metallic substance used as eye shadow. The curious evolution of the word seems to have come as distilled spirits were used to prepare the cosmetic. Then the word use changed from the metallic tint itself to the ethanol-based vehicle. Eventually a fluid produced by distillation came to be called alcohol.

The modern Arabic word for **alcohol,** *al kuhool,* is best translated as "demon" or "spirit"; the former is a reasonable description of the effect alcohol can have. It probably reentered the Arab language from the West.

The Story of the Magic Hairball

Yet another word arising in the Middle East is **bezoar**, from medieval Arabic *badizhar*, and that word was derived from the earlier Persian *podzahr*, combining *pad*, "against," with *zahr*, "poison." Thus the bezoar was highly valued as a magical shield against plague, pox, and other communicable diseases of the time (Kennett, p. 16). But what exactly was a bezoar, and where did it come from?

The legendary bezoar was a ball of hair and undigested food found in the stomach or intestines of animals, the site varying with the author you read (Fig. 4.8). Haubrich (p. 29) is very specific as to the source, describing it as "the hair ball extracted from the rectum of a wild Asiatic mountain goat." Arab apothecaries brought the bezoar to Europe, and eventually the word was used to describe various amulets: the **bezoar of Sol** (gold), **bezoar of Luna** (silver), and **bezoar of Saturn**

Fig. 4.7 A 1973 photo of
a then-legal hashish shop
in Kathmandu, Nepal.
Credit: Roger McLassus.
Creative Commons https://
commons.wikimedia.org/
wiki/File:Hashish-shop-
Kathmandu-1973.jpg

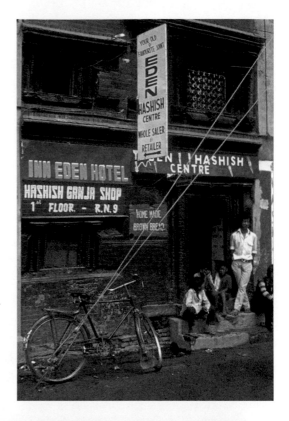

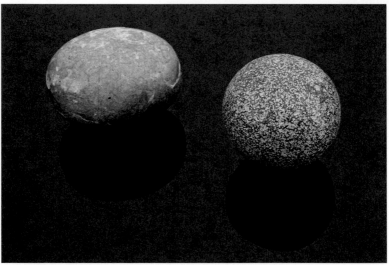

Fig. 4.8 A bezoar stone from a camel (*left*) compared with 45 mm stone (*right*). Source: Wellcome Images. Creative Commons. https://commons.wikimedia.org/wiki/File:Spherical_bezoar_stone_ from_unknown_animal,_1551-1750_Wellcome_L0058457.jpg

(lead). **Bezoar stones** were sometimes added to drinks to counteract any poison added by an assassin.

Today we no longer use magic hairballs to protect against poison or disease. But we do occasionally encounter a bezoar in a human patient. One is the **phytobezoar**, from Greek *phyton*, meaning "plant," occurring in persons eating indigestible fibers from plants such as persimmons. In other cases, clinicians occasionally encounter **trichobezoars**, from Greek *trichos*, meaning "hair," in individuals who pluck out and swallow their own hair. The compulsion to ingest one's own hair has been called the **Rapunzel syndrome**, named for the fairy tale by the Brothers Grimm about a beautiful maiden in a tower whose hair grew long enough to allow the prince to climb to her. The condition is also called **trichophagia**.

The Red Boys of the Gold Coast

Severe dietary deficiency can result in **kwashiorkor**. Dirckx (p. 70) tells that in the language of Ghana, the word means "disease of the deposed child," meaning an illness a baby suffers when a new baby comes. Also, being orphaned or otherwise abandoned in a developing country can certainly lead to very poor nutrition.

On the other hand, Durham (p. 306) writes that on the African Gold Coast, kwashiorkor means "red boy." This is also probably an appropriate term: The disease characteristically causes depigmentation of the skin and hair, and in Africa, these children may appear "red." Kwashiorkor also causes lassitude, mental apathy, anemia, diarrhea, and retarded growth. Hypoalbuminemia and fatty hepatic enlargement lead to the swollen abdomen typically found. If untreated, many children with kwashiorkor die of the disease (Fig. 4.9).

The disease was first described in 1933 by Jamaican physician Cicely Williams (1893–1992), working in Ghana. She described kwashiorkor occurring in infants with a diet specifically lacking protein. Later in Malaya, she campaigned against the substitution of sweetened condensed milk for mothers' milk in feeding newborn infants.

Black Fever and the Sand Fly

A common name for **visceral leishmaniasis** is **kala-azar**, which means "black fever" in Hindi. It is a disease of poverty, famine, and high population density, occurring in many areas worldwide, including East Africa and the Indian subcontinent. The cause is a protozoan parasite, *L. donovani*, spread by the sand fly. If untreated, the mortality rate with kala-azar is devastatingly high.

The allusion to "black fever" comes from blackening of the skin, seen originally in patients in India, but this manifestation is often not present, sometimes leading to delay in diagnosis.

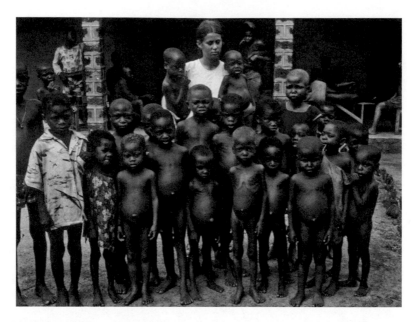

Fig. 4.9 Kwashiorkor in children in a Nigerian orphanage, 1960. Note the swollen bellies, and four of the children have depigmented gray-blond hair. Centers for Disease Control and Prevention. Public Domain. https://commons.wikimedia.org/wiki/File:Kwashiorkor_6903.jpg

The parasitic agent of kala-azar was discovered by Irish physician Charles Donovan (1863–1951), working in the Indian Medical Service. Donovan published his findings in 1903. At this time, working independently, Scottish doctor William Boog Leishman (1865–1926) also discovered the parasite and also published his work in 1903. Because of the virtually simultaneous publications describing the organism, it was named *Leishmania donovani*, honoring both men.

In an interesting twist, however, Leishman first discovered the parasite in the spleen of a soldier while working in Dum Dum, a town near Calcutta, India. He called the illness **Dumdum fever**.

The Tale of the Dangerous Bug

The disease caused by *Orientia tsutsugamushi*, first identified in Japan in 1930, is called **scrub typhus**, **bush typhus**, or **tsutsugamushi fever**. The organism was originally classified as part of the *Rickettsia* genus, but has been reclassified as in the *Orientia* genus of the family Rickettsiaceae. The word **tsutsugamushi** comes from Japanese *tsutsuga*, meaning "sickness," and *mushi*, "insect."

Mites, also known as "chiggers," typically found in areas of dense scrub vegetation, spread the organism. There is an interesting gender difference in those with the disease. In Korea, female patients with **tsutsugamushi fever** outnumber males, but not in Japan, perhaps related to the differing gender roles in the two countries, with Korean women more likely to do agricultural work where they would encounter mites.

Scrub typhus played a role in World War II, causing many casualties during jungle warfare in New Guinea, prompting the use of DDT to combat mites and ticks near Allied bases.

Bringing Home the Tattoo

The patient with a **tattoo** may come to the physician seeking removal, and then the indelible marking of the skin becomes a medical issue. Tattoo comes from *tatau*, meaning "mark," in the Polynesian language. Although previously known in the Western world, in 1769, Captain James Cook (1728–1779) and his crew popularized the practice when they brought home both the word and some examples of brightly colored skin markings (Evans, p. 1064). Joseph Banks (1743–1820), a naturalist sailing with Cook on the *HMS Endeavor*, described in his journal the tattoos observed in the indigenous peoples of Polynesia; Banks himself returned tattooed.

Today a tattoo is acquired for one of many reasons: a pledge of love, a symbol of religious devotion, a souvenir of an important event, a permanent enhancement of eyebrows, or as eyeliner (Fig. 4.10). Physicians may employ tattooing to conceal areas of vitiligo and to mask a surgical scar. Alzheimer patients have received tattoos to be used for identification in case of wandering. Some commercial enterprises have even paid individuals to have their logos permanently emblazoned on their skin, so-called skinvertising.

Running Amok or Amuck

We don't often hear the term **run amok** (or **amuck**) used in conversation anymore, but it was used more commonly a generation or two ago to describe an uninhibited violent eruption. The disease **amok** is described by Magalini (p. 29): "Homicidal attack, preceded by period of depression, preoccupation. In an unprovoked outburst of rage the patient runs about armed, usually with a knife, and attacks indiscriminately any person or animal that he encounters before he is overpowered or kills himself."

The word **amok** is a direct appropriation of the Malay word meaning "bloody attack" or "impulse to murder." The index population is males of the Maori tribes of New Zealand. Ciardi (p. 7) suggests that the frenzy may be related to use of a hallucinogenic mushroom. There was a cultural belief that an evil tiger spirit had entered the body, causing the rampage, and thus survivors of amok were forgiven for their deeds. The condition was encountered in 1770 by British Captain James Cook on an around-the-world voyage.

Fig. 4.10 The tattooed
woman, by Henri de
Toulouse-Lautrec
(1864–1901). Public
Domain. https://commons.
wikimedia.org/wiki/
File:Lautrec_the_tattooed_
woman_1894.jpg

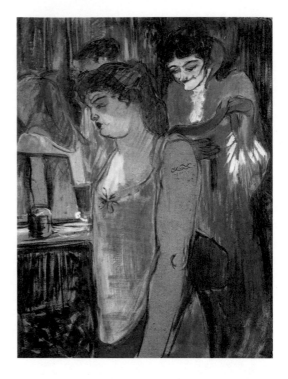

As was the case in the sixteenth and seventeenth centuries, words often had several spellings. Amok sometimes was written amuck, and both versions are found in today's dictionaries.

Agar, Dessert, and Jelly

A favorite ingredient in Asian desserts, **agar** is a gelatinous substance derived from seaweed. Credit for its discovery circa 1658 goes to Japanese innkeeper Mino Tarōzaemon, who named the substance *kanten* in Japanese. The name agar comes from *agar-agar*, the Malaysian name for jelly.

Then in 1882, German scientist Walther Hesse (1846–1911) was working as an assistant in the laboratory of German microbiologist Robert Koch (1843–1910), the latter known for his pioneering work on infectious diseases and his identification of the organisms causing cholera and tuberculosis. As the story goes, while on a picnic with his wife Angelina (Lina), Hesse observed that her jellies resisted melting in the summer heat. Why? Lina replied that they were made of agar, a method she had learned from a neighbor who had recently emigrated from Indonesia. Hesse took the idea back to the laboratory, where he found that agar could be used as a culture medium for bacteria.

Today, in the microbiology laboratory, we have the **agar plate**, a Petri dish (see Chap. 7) containing agar plus assorted nutrients, which is used to grow bacteria and other microorganisms.

The Perils of Polished Rice

A nutritional deficiency encountered in countries where polished rice is the dietary staple, **beriberi** is caused by an inadequate intake of vitamin B1, **thiamin**. The disease name is a Singhalese word meaning "weak." The word duplication, a device often seen in Eastern languages (see agar-agar, above), is used for emphasis. Thus, **beriberi** means not only weak but extremely weak. Related thiamine deficiency diseases are **Wernicke encephalopathy** and **Korsakoff syndrome**. How was the beriberi-thiamine connection discovered?

Credit for elucidating the cause of beriberi goes to Dutch physician Christiaan Eijkman (1858–1930), working in the Dutch East Indies (Fig. 4.11). For a long time, beriberi, like scurvy, had plagued the crews of ships on long voyages. The end of the nineteenth century was a time when physicians and scientists were heady with the discoveries of Pasteur and Koch regarding microorganisms and communicable diseases; beriberi must surely be one of these. Eijkman worked first with rabbits, injecting them with diseased blood, but achieved inconsequential results. Then, because they were less expensive, Eijkman switched to the use of chickens in his experiments.

Without any scientific intervention, his chickens developed beriberi and later, just as mysteriously, they recovered. Eijkman learned that, shortly before the chickens became sick, his assistant had begun feeding the chickens surplus cooked polished rice from the military hospital kitchen, rice that we now know is thiamine-deficient. Then a new cook in the military kitchen forbade feeding "military" rice to "civilian" birds, and the chickens, now consuming unpolished rice, recovered. In the years to come, Eijkman, working with colleague Adolphe Vorderman (1844–1902), continued research on chickens, and then on humans, showing the connection between diet and beriberi. Eijkman's work eventually earned him the 1929 Nobel Prize in Physiology or Medicine, shared with Sir Frederick Gowland Hopkins (1861–1947) for Hopkins' "discovery of the growth-stimulating vitamins" [4].

In a sad twist of fate, Cicely Williams, who described kwashiorkor (see above) as a nutritional deficiency in children in Africa, developed beriberi. She was in Malaya at the time of the Japanese invasion in 1941, fled to Singapore, and, when this city fell, was imprisoned for 4 years. During this time, consuming a vitamin-deficient starvation diet, she developed beriberi, leaving her with permanent peripheral neuropathy.

Four decades after Eijkman's work, in 1937, the name for vitamin B1, **thiamin**, was first proposed by American chemist Robert R. Williams (1886–1965), combining Greek *theion*, "sulfur," with "amine." Thiamin is described chemically as an organosulfur compound.

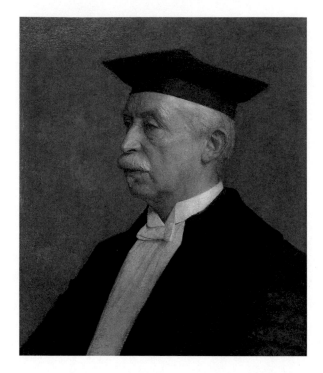

Fig. 4.11 Christiaan
Eijkman (1858–1930).
Author: Jan Veth. Public
Domain. https://commons.
wikimedia.org/wiki/
File:Christiaan_Eijkman,_
portret_door_Jan_Pieter_
Veth,_1923.jpg

The Laughing Death Syndrome

The medical name of the **laughing death syndrome** is **kuru**. The word comes from the language of the Fore tribe of Papua New Guinea, to whom the disease seems to be restricted. The disease is a transmissible and incurable degenerative neurological disorder, caused by a prion, as is classic Creutzfeldt–Jakob disease.

Manifestations of kuru begin with a tremor, followed by loss of coordination and incapacitation. The hallmark of the disease is uncontrolled, inappropriate, and almost continuous laughter. Death within 3–6 months is typical of the full-blown disease.

Although Durham (p. 305) postulates a hereditary disposition, the more likely cause is "mortuary cannibalism." The bodies of victims of kuru, including the brains, were consumed in a ritualistic fashion. According to Costandi, "Those that died of kuru were highly regarded as sources of food, because they had layers of fat which resembled pork. It was primarily the Fore women who took part in this ritual. Often they would feed morsels of brain to young children and elderly relatives. Among the tribe, it was, therefore, women, children, and the elderly who most often became infected" [5].

Cocaine: From the Jungle of Peru to the Halls of Academe in Baltimore

First isolated in 1860 in the laboratory of German chemist Friedrich Wöhler (1800–1882), and named by him **cocaine**, the drug had been used for centuries by indigenous peoples of South America, notably Peru and Bolivia. The natives of the Andes Mountains combated fatigue by chewing leaves of the *Erythroxylum coca* plant. **Coca** and **cocaine** come from the word *cuca* in the Quechua language of the South American Andes (Fig. 4.12).

Its legitimate medical use began in 1884 when Austrian ophthalmologist Karl Koller (1857–1944) demonstrated the value of cocaine as an anesthetic in eye surgery, earning him the sobriquet "Coca Koller." But use of the drug was to take a more "recreational" turn, championed by Austrian neurologist Sigmund Freud (1856–1939) (Fig. 4.11). In 1884, at age 28, after experimenting with cocaine, Freud wrote to his fiancé, Martha Bernays:

> Woe to you, my princess, when I come. I will kiss you quite hard and feed you until you are plump. And if you willfully resist, you shall see who is the stronger, a gentle little girl who doesn't eat enough, or a big wild man with cocaine in his body. In my last depression I took coca again and a small dose lifted me to the heights in a wonderful fashion. I am busy collecting the literature for a song of praise to this wonderful substance. (Li, p. 209)

Fig. 4.12 Cocaine powder. Public Domain. https:// commons.wikimedia.org/ wiki/File:Cocaine3.jpg

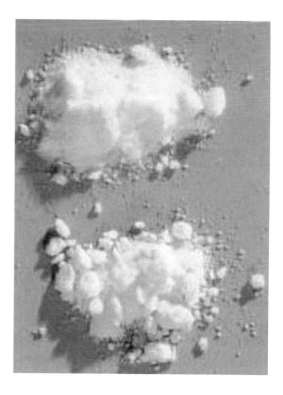

Freud went on to publish his "song of praise," *Über Coca*, later that year.

The next chapter in our cocaine story takes place at Baltimore, Maryland. Surgeon William Halsted was one of the "Big Four" founders (another was Sir William Osler) of Johns Hopkins University School of Medicine; he was the first US surgeon to perform a radical mastectomy for breast cancer. He read Freud's paper and experimented with the drug. Halsted eventually became addicted to cocaine, and also later to morphine, which continued throughout his professional life, an "open secret" at the hospital during his time there (Taylor, 2016, p. 272) .

Quinine

Another word from the Peruvian Quechua language is **quinine**, long used as an antimalarial drug. The word in the indigenous language is *kina*, meaning "bark of a tree," later evolving to *quina*. Swedish botanist Carl Linnaeus (1707–1778) named the genus of trees yielding healing bark *Cinchona*, honoring the Second Countess of Chinchón, whose malaria was cured by the bark of a native tree. Some doubt this attribution, but it is a good tale. One special bark came from the "fever tree," now classified as *Cinchona calisaya* (Fig. 4.13).

English physician Thomas Sydenham (1624–1689), sometimes dubbed "the English Hippocrates," described the malarial fevers of his time and helped promote the use of Peruvian bark as therapy (Garrison, p. 270).

In the 1570s, Jesuit priests brought **Peruvian bark** to Europe, and in the seventeenth century, it was used to treat malaria in Rome, which at that time was surrounded by mosquito-infested swamps. In preparation for his historic exploration of the Louisiana Territory beginning in 1804, Meriwether Lewis spent one-third of his medical supply budget—all of 30 dollars—on **Peruvian bark**. Quinine remained the drug of choice for malaria until the 1940s, when newer, more effective drugs began to replace it. During World War II, American scientist Edwin H. Land (1909–1991), inventor of the Polaroid Land Camera, contributed to the war effort by leading a research team that discovered how to produce synthetic quinine. The drug is no longer considered first-line therapy for malaria.

But what began as the bark of a Peruvian tree has not disappeared from our lives. We still find quinine as an ingredient in "tonic water." During the time of the British Raj in India (1858–1947), soldiers were required to take a daily dose of quinine to prevent malaria. They masked the bitter taste of quinine with distilled spirits, giving us the popular combination, gin and tonic.

Of Courage and Chopped Liver

Old English, spoken in England from the fifth to the twelfth century, was the language of the Anglo-Saxons, with a strong Germanic influence. Several modern medical words come from Old English, such as *lifer*, meaning **liver**, the large, multifunction organ in the right upper quadrant of the abdomen.

Fig. 4.13 Cinchona calisaya plant. Credit: Franz Eugen Köhler. Public Domain. https:// commons.wikimedia.org/ wiki/File:Cinchona_ calisaya_-_Köhler–s_ Medizinal-Pflanzen-179. jpg

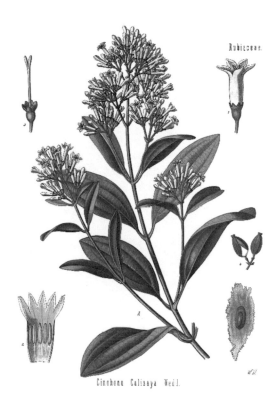

The liver is the only internal organ that can regenerate tissue. This characteristic of the organ supports the Greek myth of Prometheus who, as punishment by the Gods for giving mortals the secret of fire, was chained to a rock and suffered having his liver devoured by a vulture each day, only to replace itself overnight.

In Plato's time (ca 428–347 BCE), the liver was believed to be the site of wrath and jealousy Late, during medieval times, the organ was thought to be an organ of courage; one who acted in a cowardly manner was "lily-livered."

Today we have the phrase, "What am I, chopped liver?" The origin of this remark is little murky, but the best answer is this: Chopped liver, not very appetizing, is always a side dish, never a main dish. Thus to be "chopped liver" is to be minimized, overlooked, or, as my grandchildren might say, "dissed."

Little Spots and High Fevers

According to the Oxford English Dictionary, Middle English describes the English language spoken from the middle of the twelfth century until 1500. At that time *maseles*, the plural of *masel*, meant "little spots." Today we use the word **measles**,

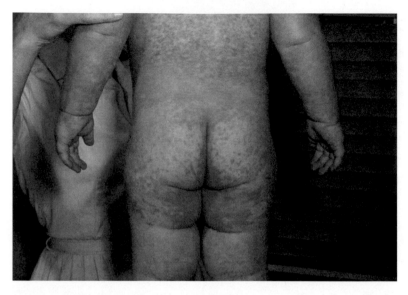

Fig. 4.14 The rash of measles. Centers for Disease Control and Prevention. Public Domain. https://commons.wikimedia.org/wiki/File:Measles_rash_PHIL_4497_lores.jpg

although we don't see the disease much anymore. We forget that prior to the introduction of the measles vaccine in 1963, measles was considered one of the "usual childhood diseases."

Measles, with the clinical name **rubeola**, may have been common, but it was not necessarily a benign disease. The viral infection causes cough, red eyes, nasal congestion, and high fever, often exceeding 104 °F. **Koplik spots**, small white dots sometimes seen in the mouth and considered pathognomonic for the disease, are named for American pediatrician Henry Koplik (1858–1927), who described the lesions in 1896. A red maculopapular rash comes a few days after initial symptoms (Fig. 4.14). Measles complications, occurring more often than many realize, may include pneumonia, blindness, and encephalitis.

Until the early tenth century, there was widespread confusion about the spotted diseases: measles, **smallpox**, and **chickenpox**. The first clear description of measles was written by Persian physician Rhazes (860–932). His monograph *The Book of Smallpox and Measles* was the first to distinguish between the two diseases.

Despite all we know of the risks involved, there are still parents who refuse to have their children immunized against measles. As recently as 2015, there was an outbreak of measles that started at Disneyland in California and spread to several US states, Mexico, and Canada. In this outbreak, 147 persons were confirmed with the disease, but there were no deaths [6].

Rickets

The word **rickets**, describing a disease characterized by severe softening of the bones, comes directly from a dialect of the English language, called West Country English, spoken in Dorset, Somerset, and nearby counties in the seventeenth century. In fact, the English word may have its origins in the Greek *rachitis*, meaning "in the spine." Onions (p. 766) tells that the disease was "first observed in Dorset and Somerset." This is probably not precisely accurate.

Bordley and Harvey (p. 242) tell of Thersites, a bow-legged Greek soldier in the Trojan War "with rounded shoulders that almost met across his chest." They go on to describe fifteenth- and sixteenth-century paintings depicting the Christ child with bowed legs and chest deformities characteristic of rickets. English physician Daniel Whistler (1619–1684) provided the first systematic description of the disease in 1645.

Today rickets is rarely encountered in the developed world, although infants fed plant-based milk substitutes without vitamin D supplementation are at risk. On the other hand, rickets is still sometimes seen in children in developing countries (Fig. 4.15) .

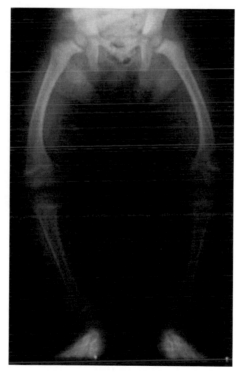

Fig. 4.15 Anteroposterior (AP) view of the legs in a 2-year-old child with rickets. Credit: Michael L. Richardson, M.D. Sept 28th, 2004. Creative Commons. https://commons.wikimedia.org/wiki/File:XrayRicketsLegssmall.jpg

References

1. Centers for Disease Control and Prevention. Sexually transmitted diseases. Available at: http://www.cdc.gov/std/syphilis/stdfact-syphilis-detailed.htm
2. Karlen A. A capsule history of medical nostrums. Physician's World. 1974;11(7):59.
3. Jamieson HC. Catechism in medical history. Can. Med Assn J. 1944;51:376.
4. Allchin D. Christiaan Eijkman and the cause of beriberi. Available at: https://www1.umn.edu/ships/modules/biol/Christian%20Eijkman%20&%20Beriberi.pdf
5. Costandi M. Mad cows, cannibalism and the shaking death. Available at: https://www.the-guardian.com/science/neurophilosophy/2013/sep/26/mad-cows-cannibalism-kuru
6. Phadke VK. Association between vaccine refusal and vaccine-preventable diseases in the United States: a review of measles and pertussis. JAMA. 2016:315:1149.

Chapter 5
Medical Words Linked to Places

Diseases named after places are **toponymous diseases**, from the Greek *topos*, meaning "place," and *onoma*, "name." Toponymous diseases may take their names from towns, rivers, islands, forests, mountains, valleys, countries, continents, and even trenches dug in the ground. Sometimes we can track the person who connected the place with the disease and created the name; more often what the disease was and is called simply arose within the local culture.

There are examples of **toponymous diseases** from virtually every part of the world. A group of enteroviruses first isolated from a patient in a small community in the Hudson Valley of New York State takes its name from the town—the **Coxsackie viruses**. **Tularemia** was named by American epidemiologist Edward Francis (1872–1957) in 1919 to memorialize Tulare County, in California, USA, combining the county name with the Greek *haima*, meaning "blood." In 1928, the virus causing **Ross River Fever**, a disease affecting both humans and kangaroos, was discovered in a mosquito collected near the Ross River in New South Wales, Australia. A tick-borne disease hosted by muskrats and water voles was named for the city in southwestern Siberia, Russia, where it was first found in the 1940s—**Omsk hemorrhagic fever**. **Katayama fever**, formally known as acute systemic schistoso-miasis, was named for the place where it was originally reported, the Katayama River Valley in Japan.

In 2015, the World Health Organization (WHO) declared what they called "best practices for naming new human infectious diseases." Citing "unintended negative impacts by stigmatizing certain communities or economic sectors," the WHO decried names such as swine flu, Rift Valley fever, and Middle East respiratory syndrome. They also condemn the use of people's names, such as Creutzfeldt–Jakob disease and Chagas disease. The directive goes on to point out that the guidelines apply only to newly recognized diseases and syndromes, and not to disease names already described [1].

I can understand the sensitivities of Coxsackie town residents, the inhabitants of the Rift Valley, all who live in the Middle East, and maybe even swine. But to forbid future disease nomenclature based on places will be one more loss of the richness of our amazing medical language.

In this chapter, I will begin with the current major concerns—the viral diseases causing today's outbreaks, epidemics, and pandemics. I will then present disease names linked to a variety of places, ending with those in Europe and America.

Cars and Forests and Summer Olympics

In 2016, Indian automobile manufacturer Tata Motors decided not to call its new hatchback car by its planned name Zica, derived from "Zippy Car." This is just one more reaction to the epidemic of **Zika virus** infections that the World Health Organization has declared a global emergency (Fig. 5.1). In addition to causing fever and malaise, when the patient is pregnant, the Zika virus may also cause birth defects, notably **microcephaly** (from Greek words meaning "small" and "head"). Some adult Zika virus patients go on to develop the Guillain–Barré syndrome. The Zika virus has been a dark cloud over the fragile economy of Brazil in many ways, including its adverse impact on attendance at the 2016 Rio de Janeiro Summer Olympic Games.

The Zika virus is, for most of the world, a newcomer. On New Year's Day 2015, for example, hardly anyone had heard of the infection. Now the disease is well known, but where did it arise and how did it get its unusual name?

In the 1940s, researchers identified a transmissible agent in the blood removed earlier from a rhesus macaque laboratory monkey sick with a fever. The monkey had come from a mosquito-infested jungle in Uganda called the Zika Forest, the name coming from the word for "overgrown" in the Luganda language of Uganda.

Fig. 5.1 Symptoms of Zika virus. Credit: Beth. herlin. Creative Commons. https://commons. wikimedia.org/wiki/ File:ZIKA.png

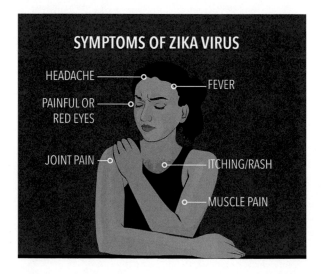

From here, and only in the past few years, the virus has migrated across Asia and the Pacific to Central and South America, reaching pandemic proportions in some areas. In addition to mosquito-borne infection, we now have discovered sexually transmitted Zika virus disease and continue to learn more each year.

Another Virus from Uganda

One might assume that the **West Nile virus** came from Egypt, but in fact, the organism was first discovered in the West Nile district of Uganda in 1937. This mosquito-transmitted arbovirus was considered a problem only for birds and horses until the 1990s, when human infections began to be reported. Most West Nile viral infections are subclinical, but a few are complicated by meningoencephalitis and a flaccid paralysis reminiscent of polio.

The West Nile virus is a member of the family *Flaviviridae*, from the Latin *flavus*, meaning "yellow." The family was named for the **yellow fever virus**, which tends to cause liver damage, giving its victims a yellow jaundiced appearance (Fig. 5.2).

Other Viral Causes of Encephalitis

Viruses of the *Flaviviridae* family have turned up in various places and have often acquired the names of those locations. **Japanese encephalitis** is a disease of domestic pigs and birds, notably herons, that can be spread to humans by mosquitoes. It is the chief cause of viral encephalitis in Asia.

Fig. 5.2 Electron micrograph of the West Nile virus. Centers for disease control and prevention. Public Domain. https://commons. wikimedia.org/wiki/ File:West_Nile_virus_ EM_PHIL_2290_lores.jpg

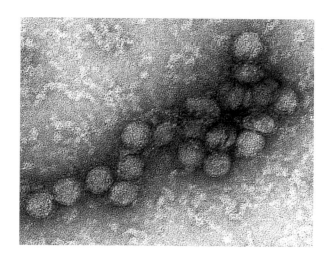

Another member of the *Flaviviridae* family is *Mansonia pseudotitillans*, the cause of **Saint Louis encephalitis**. The mosquito-borne disease harkens to 1933 in St. Louis, Missouri, when more than a thousand cases were reported.

La Crosse encephalitis is caused by a virus from the family *Bunyaviridae*, the same family that causes **Crimean–Congo hemorrhagic fever**. Discovered in the early 1960s in La Crosse, Wisconsin, the mosquito-transmitted disease is found chiefly in the Midwestern and Appalachian regions of the United States.

Homes of the Hemorrhagic Fevers

Several families of RNA virus can cause hemorrhagic fevers. The **hantavirus** takes its name from the place where the virus was first isolated in the late 1970s: the Hantaan River valley in South Korea. Rodents, such as the cotton rat, spread the hantavirus, and humans acquire the virus through contact with rodent feces, urine, or saliva. The hantavirus belongs to the family *Bunyaviridae*.

Lassa virus, a member of the *Arenaviridae* family, causes **Lassa hemorrhagic fever**. The disease was initially described in 1969 in Lassa, a town in Borno State, Nigeria. A zoonotic disease, the reservoir is rodents, notably multimammate mice (*Mastomys natalensis*), whose excreta—feces and urine—can be aerosolized, and the disease can be spread by inhalation of these tiny particles.

Two members of the family *Filoviridae* are the **Ebola virus** and the **Marburg virus**. **Ebola hemorrhagic fever**, spread among humans by direct contact with body fluids, such as blood, semen, or breast milk, of an infected individual, causes death by internal and external bleeding in approximately half of infected persons. The name Ebola comes from the Ebola River, which flows near the village of Yambuku in the Democratic Republic of the Congo (previously Zaire), where the disease was identified in 1976 (Fig. 5.3).

The name Marburg virus did not originate in Africa, but in Germany. In the 1960s, several monkeys were sent from Uganda to Europe for use in laboratory experiments. Unknown to the scientists involved, these monkeys carried a *Filoviridae* virus, resulting in infections in several dozen researchers in three cities, including the university town of Marburg, giving the organism the name it carries today.

Of Coughs and Camels

One of the disease names specifically criticized by the WHO is the **Middle East respiratory syndrome (MERS)**. The term "Middle East" may not have the exotic flavor of a river in South Korea or a forest in Uganda, but it does give a good indication of where the disease began, and a hint as to why it was first noted in this part of the world.

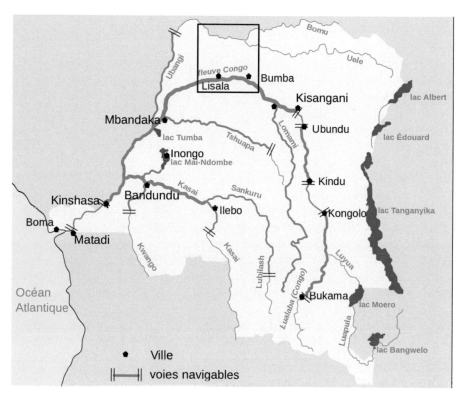

Fig. 5.3 The Congo River basin with the Ebola River region indicated by the square. Credit: Fleuve rdc.svg: Aliesin; Derivative work: Miguelferig. Creative Commons. https://commons.wiki-media.org/wiki/File:Fleuve_rdc_with_Ebola_region_indicated.svg

MERS, first reported in Saudi Arabia in 2012, is a viral disease of the respiratory tract causing cough, fever, dyspnea, and sometimes death. Only a few cases have been reported in the United States, and, so far, these have been contracted during travel in the Middle East and imported by returning travelers. Other cases have been reported in more than two dozen countries including Great Britain, Germany, Greece, Korea, China, Malaysia, and the Philippines.

The intriguing aspect of MERS is the likely connection to camels. The causative virus (MERS-CoV) has been found in camels, and some patients with the disease have told of contact with camels. The WHO warns against drinking raw camel milk or camel urine or eating undercooked camel meat. So perhaps the "Middle East" part of the disease name is on target. Where else but the Middle East do humans live in close communion with camels? And drinking camel urine? Yes, some in the region believe that drinking camel urine has medicinal value.

The Middle Eastern Origin of the Word Vitamin

What could be the connection between the **vitamins** essential to our health, a Polish biochemist, and camel dung in the Middle East? The story goes back more than three millennia.

As early as the Eighteenth Dynasty (c. 1543–1292 BCE and the time of King Tutankhamun), the early Egyptians worshiped the god *Amun*, also called *Amun-Ra* or *Ammon*, as the leading god of the Empire, later to be identified with the Greek god Zeus (Fig. 5.4). In what is now Libya, they built a temple to Ammon where Egyptians came to worship their god; while they did so, their camels fertilized the nearby sand with urine and feces. It was from this sand that *sal ammoniac*, the "salt of Ammon," was first derived. In fact, the ancient Greek word for "sand" is *ammos*, probably related to the name of the god (Shipley, p. 20).

From *sal ammoniac* comes **ammonia** (NH3), a pungent-smelling, colorless gas, so named in 1782 by Swedish Chemist Torbern Bergman (1735–1784), and from ammonia comes our word **amine. Amines** are derived from ammonia by chemical substitution of one or more of the hydrogen atoms with other radicals.

The next etymologic landmark in the story of the word vitamin came in 1912 when Polish biochemist Casimir Funk (1884–1967) introduced the concept of **amines** as being vital to life. He postulated that there were at least four necessary

Fig. 5.4 Amun statuette with shuti feathers, from Thebes. 19th–20th dynasty. Credit: Einsamer Schütze. Creative Commons. https://commons.wikimedia.org/wiki/File:Statuette_of_Amun_Hildesheim.jpg

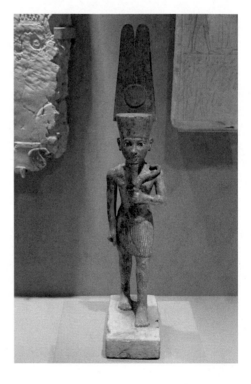

amines and that without them patients would develop beriberi, scurvy, rickets, and/ or pellagra. To form his word, Funk combined –*amine* with the Latin word for life, *vita* (recall the 1960 Fellini movie, *La Dolce Vita*—the "sweet life"). Funk's original word *vitamine* was later shortened to *vitamin* when it was learned that not all vitamins contained amines [2].

Casimir Funk was nominated for a Nobel Prize in 1914, 1925, 1926, and 1946. He never received the award.

Today we have vitamins A, B (a number of these), C, D, E, and K, the latter so designated because of its action in coagulation (originally named *koagulationsvitamin* in German). There are also vitamin wannabes, such as the bogus cancer drug amygdalin (Laetrile), a cyanogenic substance found in apricot kernels and dubbed **vitamin B17**, perhaps alluding to the World War II Flying Fortress.

We have come a long way from camel urine to drugstore shelves full of colorful vitamin bottles and a few misbegotten imitators.

The Skull from the Mountains

In Chap. 2, I told of Prometheus chained by Zeus for giving humans the gift of fire; the location where he was restrained was the Caucasus Mountains near what are now Iran and Turkey (Fig. 5.5). It was in these mountains that German scientist Johann Friedrich Blumenbach (1752–1840) discovered a skull. Blumenbach,

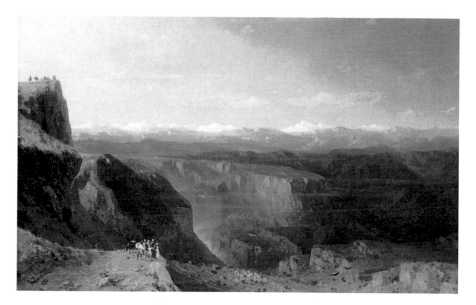

Fig. 5.5 The Caucasus Mountains. Oil on canvas, by Ivan Aivazovsky (1817–1900). Public Domain. https://commons.wikimedia.org/wiki/File:Aivasovsky_Ivan_Constantinovich_The_Caucasus.jpg

considered the father of physical anthropology, suggested that the various human subspecies ("races") could be classified by the study of their skulls.

Based on his anthropometric comparisons, in 1781, he proposed five families of humans: yellow (Mongolians), black (Ethiopians), red (American Indians), brown (Malaysians), and white. For the name of this last category, he used the location of the finest skull of all, the Caucasus Mountains, and from that moment on, white persons became **Caucasian** (Gershen, p. 113).

The Island of Female Homosexuality

It started with the Greek lyric poet Sappho (ca. 620–570 BCE). She was born on the island of **Lesbos**, located in the Aegean Sea off the west coast of Turkey and a center of civilization even before the Golden Age of Greece in the fifth century BCE. She was the most renowned poetess of her day, and her lines had a distinctive "Sapphic meter." Sappho shared her poetry with a cohort of young women, and probably because of the erotic passion of some of her poems, the tale has evolved regarding homosexual relationships between the poetess and her students. Thus female homosexuality came to be named for the island, Lesbos, and a female homosexual, wherever she lived, became a **lesbian.**

A word less often used to describe women who love other women is **Sapphism**, a synonym for **lesbianism**. In fact, according to Hendrickson (p. 120), Sappho was probably married and had a son, although many will argue that this would not be solid evidence of her sexual preferences.

Malta Fever in the Crimean War

The Crimean War was fought in the mid-1850s between Russia and an alliance of the United Kingdom, France, and Turkey. It was the war that gave us Florence Nightingale and the Charge of the Light Brigade. During this war British medical officers on the island of Malta noticed a disease characterized by sweating, joint and muscle pains, and a fluctuating fever. A logical name for the mysterious malady was **Malta fever**.

In 1861, British medical officer Jeffrey Allen Marston (1831–1911) described his personal experience with the disease, and in 1887, Scottish microbiologist David Bruce (1855–1931) linked the disease to an organism that came to be called *Brucella abortus*. The "Bruce" in the name of the genus honored Bruce; the species designation *abortus* reflects the tendency of the disease to cause abortions in cattle.

The disease was briefly called **Bang's disease**, after Danish veterinarian Bernhard Bang identified *B. abortus* as the agent causing cattle to abort. Because of the wavelike nature of the fever, the disease acquired the name **undulant fever**. Other names enjoyed popularity in various settings: **Scottish delight**, **milk sickness**, **goat fever**,

Cyprus fever, **Gibraltar fever**, and **mountain fever**. In the end, the medical and scientific communities have come to favor the name **brucellosis**, honoring the man who discerned the cause of the disease.

From a Small Town in Thessaly, Three Words

This story begins in the town of Magnesia, named for an ancient Greek tribe, the Magnetes. The town lies in the Thessaly district of Greece, an area conquered by the Romans following their victory in the Battle of Magnesia in 190 BCE, ending the Roman–Seleucid War. In this conquered area, the Romans discovered a white mineral that, applying the name of the town, they called **magnesia**. When a different substance with a dark color was found, the white substance became *Magnesia alba*, from the Latin word for "white," and the darker substance became *Magnesia nigra*, Latin for "black." In 1831, French chemist Antoine Bussy (1794–1882) found that the *Magnesia alba* yielded an element, which he named **magnesium**. *Magnesia nigra* came to be called **manganese**.

There is another twist to the **magnesium** story. In the early seventeenth century, in the town of Epsom in Surrey, England, a farmer offered his cows water from a nearby well. But the cows refused to drink. The farmer learned why when he tasted the bitter water. He also observed, however, the water seemed to heal skin abrasions and sores. The bitter-tasting substance in water came to be identified as hydrated **magnesium sulfate**, better known as **Epsom salt**. Epsom wells became a destination spa, visited by diarist and Member of Parliament Samuel Pepys; Nell Gwyn, mistress of King Charles II of England; and other seventeenth-century notables (Evans, p. 380). In the United States, there is a Magnesia Temple at the town of Sharon Springs in Schoharie County, New York (Fig. 5.6).

In addition to **Epsom salt**, **magnesium** has other medical uses: a water solution of magnesium oxide is **Milk of Magnesia**, popular as a laxative. **Magnesium** has had a role in treating ventricular arrhythmias of the heart and preeclampsia/eclampsia. It is sometimes prescribed for management of migraine or of the restless leg syndrome. And the white powder that gymnasts and weight lifters use to improve their grips is **magnesium carbonate**.

Returning to the town of Magnesia, in this region was found an iron oxide stone that had the apparently magical quality of attracting iron to itself. It was called the "Magnesian stone" and served as the source of our word **magnet** (Haubrich, p. 130).

The Little Dragon from Medina

The **Guinea worm** is a parasitic nematode that is spread when a person drinks water containing the Guinea worm larvae. The cause of the disease in humans is *Dracunculus medinensis*, and the disease is properly called **dracunculiasis**.

Fig. 5.6 The Magnesia
Temple at Sharon Springs,
New York, 2008. Credit:
Doug Kerr. Creative
Commons. https://
commons.wikimedia.org/
wiki/File:Magnesia_
Temple_Nov_08.jpg

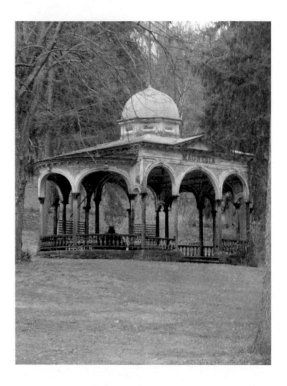

Approximately a year following ingestion of the larvae, the female Guinea worm finds its way to the skin, where it forms a blister. A little later the blister breaks and the worm begins to emerge. An adult female Guinea worm can be two to three feet long and as thick as a strand of spaghetti. Affected persons sometimes facilitate extraction of the worm by winding it around a small stick.

The name Guinea worm arose when European explorers first encountered the disease on the Guinea coast of West Africa in the seventeenth century. In Latin *Dracunculus* means "little dragon; *Dracunculus medinensis* means the "little dragon from Medina," so named because the disease was once rampant in the Muslim holy city of Medina in Saudi Arabia. Dracunculiasis is no longer endemic in either location.

The prevention of dracunculiasis requires nothing more than drinking filtered water, and the disease is on the threshold of being exterminated.

Colchicine

The source of the drug **colchicine** is the autumn crocus, *Colchicum autumnale*, so named because it was first discovered in the Colchicum region of the Republic of Georgia on the Black Sea. The plant's nickname "naked lady" refers to the

Fig. 5.7 Colchicum autumnale in the Kőszeg Mountains, Hungary. Credit: Várkonyi Tibor. Creative Commons. https://commons.wikimedia.org/wiki/File:Colchicum_autumnale2.jpg

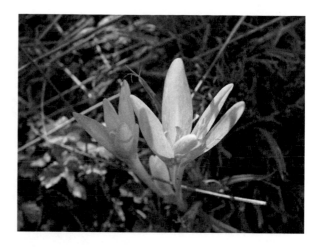

appearance of the flower without surrounding leaves. The extract of the plant can be highly toxic, and severe accidental poisonings have occurred, several involving cases in which the autumn crocus was mistaken for wild garlic (Fig. 5.7).

Use of the drug to treat joint pains can be traced to early Egyptian writings, circa 1500 BCE, found in the *Ebers Papyrus*. Therapeutic use of **colchicum extract** is mentioned in the writings of Persian physician Avicenna (980–1037) and French surgeon Ambroise Paré (1510–1590). American statesman Benjamin Franklin (1706–1790) brought the colchicum root to America from France and used it to treat his own attacks of gout.

In addition to its use in the treatment of gout, colchicine is sometimes used to treat **Behçet disease, pericarditis,** and **familial Mediterranean fever**; the latter is a hereditary disorder also known as **Armenian disease**.

Plaster of Paris

The word "plaster" in **plaster of Paris** came from Greek *emplastron*, to Latin *emplastrum*, to French *plastre*. But what about Paris?

Throughout history, various products had been used to bind wounds. French surgeon Guy de Chauliac (1300–1368), author of the seven-volume *Chirurgia Magna* in 1363, introduced the use of egg white to stiffen bandages [3]. However, the "Paris connection" came in 1852 when Dutch army surgeon Antonius Mathijsen (1805–1878) began incorporating gypsum into dressings used to immobilize fractures (Fig. 5.8). Mathijsen was not French, but the gypsum was quarried in the Montmartre section of Paris, hence the name plaster of Paris.

Fig. 5.8 Antonius
Mathijsen, who first used
what we now call plaster of
Paris. Public Domain.
https://commons.
wikimedia.org/wiki/
File:Antonius_
Mathijsen_1805-1878.jpg

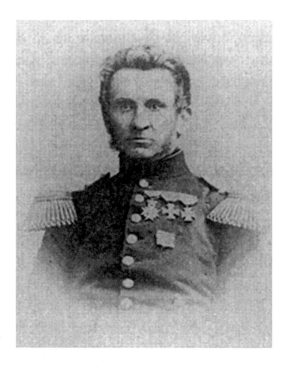

From Another Section of Paris

Although the word is probably never seen today in medical records, **clap** remains a vulgar term for gonorrhea. The common Old French term for brothel was *clapier*. The term technically translated to "rabbit burrow," and perhaps this image had something to do with the "red light" section Paris, where a number of brothels were located, being called, in the Middle Ages, *Le Clapier*. As language moved across the English Channel in the sixteenth century, *clapier* in French became clapper in English. Eventually the word was shortened to clap, generally expressed with an article as "the clap" [4].

The French had another word for this distressingly common malady, *chaude-pisse*, describing a frequent manifestation of gonorrhea. *Chaude* means "hot" in French. And *pisse*? Is translation really needed?

From a Small Danish Island

It was first called **Bramble disease** by a Norwegian physician who reported a cluster of cases of "acute muscular rheumatism" occurring in the village of Bramble in Norway. But alas, the original report and a few others that followed using the term "Bramble disease" were published only in Norwegian, and the name failed to catch on.

Then in 1933, doctoral candidate Ejnar Sylvest (1880–1972) published his thesis describing a disease outbreak on the picturesque Danish Island of **Bornholm**, in the Baltic Sea, that he termed "Bornholm disease-myalgia epidemica." Today we know this as **Bornholm disease**, as well as **epidemic pleurodynia**, **epidemic myalgia**, **devil's grip**, and **the grasp of the phantom**.

The disease causes the usual viral symptoms of fever and headache. An additional and distinguishing feature is severe pain in the lower chest, giving rise to the more colorful names of the disease. Fortunately for those with the devil's grip, the disease is self-limited and rarely fatal.

Little Red Spots and Liberty Measles

It was an American, not a German, who gave **rubella** its everyday name: **German measles**. The disease has been well known to health-care professionals and parents since first described by German physician Friedrich Hoffmann (1660–1742) in 1740. It was given the name rubella, from the Latin word meaning "little red," by English military surgeon Henry Veale in his 1866 description of an outbreak in India.

American physician J. Louis Smith coined the term "German measles" in 1874. Working at New York's Bellevue Hospital, Smith described an outbreak of the disease and, reading of similar outbreaks in Germany, he named the disease "German measles" (Bordley and Harvey, p. 657) (Fig. 5.9).

Then, amid the anti-German fervor of World War I, rubella was briefly renamed **liberty measles** (Fortuine, p. 250).

Trench Fever, Foot, and Mouth

This chapter is about diseases named for places. Is a trench a "place"? It certainly was to the World War I soldiers who spent weeks and months slogging shoulder to shoulder in deep ditches filled with icy cold water and filth. From these barely habitable ditches came the "trench" in the names of three different diseases.

The first is **trench fever**, with an estimated one million cases occurring in Western Europe during the First World War. It was first noted in an infantry private in 1915, and by 1918, the Allied General Headquarters stated: "Trench fever is a matter of national importance... and it merits the attention of every physician and pathologist who has the opportunity of working among the troops" [5].

Trench fever, caused by *Bartonella quintana* and spread by the human body louse, causes fever, prostration, a macular rash, and bone pain. Despite these manifestations, some doughboys welcomed the infection because a stay in the medical facility offered respite from the trenches. Trench fever has also been called **five-day fever**, **shin bone fever**, and **Meuse fever**; the latter is a reference to the WWI Meuse-Argonne battle of 1918. Today, we no longer have trench warfare, but we do have **urban trench fever** occurring in demented, homeless, and alcoholic persons.

Fig. 5.9 Rash of
rubella/German measles on
a child's back. Centers for
disease control and
prevention. Public Domain.
https://commons.
wikimedia.org/wiki/
File:Rash_of_rubella_on_
skin_of_child%27s_back.
JPG

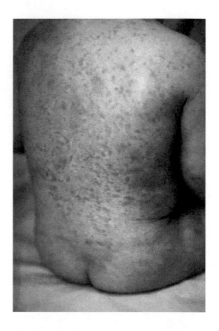

From the muddy ditches of WWI, we also get the disease name **trench foot**, describing damage to the tissues that occurs with prolonged exposure of the extremity to moist cold (Fig. 5.10). Dominique Jean Larrey (1766–1842), a surgeon in Napoleon's *Grande Armée*, noted the prevalence of what we now call **trench foot** in the French troops during their ill-fated invasion of Russia in 1812. **Trench foot** was seen not only in WWI but also in World War II and in the Vietnam War; it was called **immersion foot** or **paddy foot** in the latter jungle-based campaign.

Then there is **trench mouth**, also known as **acute necrotizing ulcerative gingivitis**, caused by a mixed bacterial infection. Recognized in Greek soldiers in the fourth century BCE, the disease was described by Scottish surgeon John Hunter (1728–1793) in 1778. At the Pasteur Institute in Paris in 1904, French physician Jean Hyacinthe Vincent (1862–1950) identified the fusospirochetal cause; one of the other names for acute necrotizing ulcerative gingivitis is **Vincent angina** [6]. In this term, *angina* reflects its true Latin meaning, "infection of the throat." The disease did not acquire the name trench mouth until World War I, when it occurred in men spending weeks and months in trenches under physical and psychological stress, receiving a poor diet, and with scant options for oral hygiene.

A Protozoan Parasite in a Popular Resort

Nantucket is a small island off Cape Cod, Massachusetts, USA. In April of 2015, the *Cape Cod Times*, in a story titled "Cape Cod a Hot Spot for Babesiosis from Ticks," reported health officials calling for "hospitals to screen blood transfusion products for babesiosis or Nantucket fever." In the article, Dr. Al DeMaria, state epidemiologist with the Massachusetts Department of Public Health, declared **Nantucket fever**

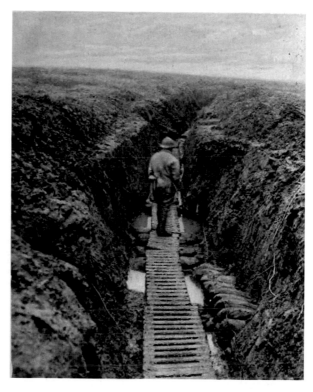

Fig. 5.10 The muddy trenches of World War I. Public Domain. https://commons.wikimedia.org/wiki/File:FrenchTrenchInMudWWI--nsillustratedwar04londuoft.jpg

to be the "No. 1 transfusion-transmitted infection" in the United States [7]. What is this toponymous disease that many health professionals have never heard of?

Nantucket fever, caused by a tick-borne protozoan parasite called *Babesia microti*, causes manifestations not unlike malaria, including fever, arthralgia, lymphadenopathy, and hemolytic anemia. The formal name for the febrile illness is **babesiosis**, first described by Romanian scientist Victor Babeş (1854–2926) as a disease of cattle and sheep. The first human case of babesiosis was reported in 1957.

In cattle, babesiosis is sometimes called **Texas cattle fever**, **tick fever**, or **red-water fever**, the latter referring to the appearance of blood in the urine. In the United States, human babesiosis has been reported chiefly in Northeastern and Midwestern states and occurs most often during warm weather.

The Dangers of the Deer Tick

If a young physician today were asked to identify a disease named for a place, the answer might well be **Lyme disease**, also called **Lyme borreliosis**. Although the disease had been recognized in Europe since the eighteenth century and documented

Fig. 5.11 Erythema
migrans, the bulls-eye rash
of Lyme disease. Centers
for disease control and
prevention. Public Domain.
https://commons.
wikimedia.org/wiki/
File:Erythema_migrans.jpg

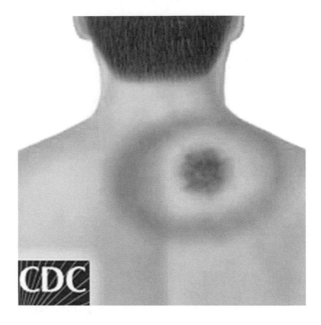

in Wisconsin in 1970, the full spectrum of the disease was not recognized until
1975, in connection with a series of cases in southeastern Connecticut, including the
small towns of Lyme and Old Lyme.

The disease is caused by *Borrelia* bacteria, notably *Borrelia burgdorferi*, and is
spread by the same vector as Nantucket fever/babesiosis: the *Ixodes* **tick**, also called
the **deer tick**. A curious, perhaps pathognomonic, feature of the disease is the early
appearance of a "bulls-eye" rash, called **erythema migrans**, although this helpful
diagnostic clue is not seen in all patients (Fig. 5.11). Later manifestations may
include fatigue, neurocognitive manifestations, disorders of heart rhythm, polyneu-
ropathy, and arthritis.

Lyme disease is the most commonly occurring tick-borne disease in Europe and
North America. In the United States, the areas of greatest prevalence are the
Northeast and Middle Atlantic states and western Wisconsin. In these locations,
woodsmen and woodswomen, beware of the deer tick.

Rocky Mountain Spotted Fever, Not Always in the Mountains

Another malady, along with Lyme disease, well known for its geographic label is
Rocky Mountain spotted fever. Also sometimes called **tick typhus** or **blue disease**, Rocky Mountain spotted fever was first recognized in 1896 in the Snake River
Valley in the Rocky Mountains of the Western United States. The disease is spread
by ticks carrying the causative organism, *Rickettsia rickettsii*, a name that seems

unnecessarily repetitive, like the name of the common black rat, *Rattus rattus*; the latter is an animal reservoir for fleas carrying the bacteria causing bubonic plague. The name of the organism redundantly honors American pathologist Howard Taylor Ricketts (1871–1910), who first isolated the pathogen that causes the disease.

A potentially fatal disease, Rocky Mountain spotted fever is the most commonly reported Rickettsial disease in the United States. Curiously, because of the epidemiologic distribution of the disease in America, you and I are at more risk of contracting Rocky Mountain spotted fever in North Carolina than we are in Colorado.

On an Island in Chesapeake Bay

First found in 1959 in a 5-year-old boy living on Tangier Island in Virginia's Chesapeake Bay, **Tangier disease** is also known as familial alpha-lipoprotein deficiency. It is a congenital disorder causing a severe deficiency of high-density lipoprotein (HDL) in the blood. In addition to abnormal serum lipids found on laboratory analysis, patients with Tangier disease may have splenomegaly, hepatomegaly, neuropathy, atherosclerosis, and cloudiness of the corneas of the eyes (Fig. 5.12).

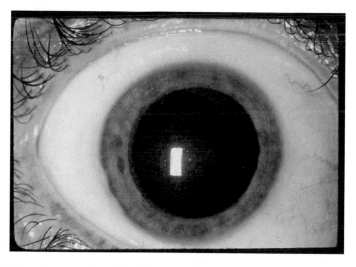

Fig. 5.12 Diffuse hazy opacity of the right cornea in the patient with Tangier disease. National Eye Institute. Public Domain. https://commons.wikimedia.org/wiki/File:Tanger.gif

Names from Cities, Countries, and Continents

There is a long list of other medical entities that came from cities, countries, and even continents. In 1960, scientists working in the city of Philadelphia, Pennsylvania, discovered the **Philadelphia chromosome**, an abnormality of chromosome 22 associated with chronic myelogenous leukemia.

Milltown, New Jersey, originally named for a local gristmill, was the manufacturing site of the anxiolytic drug **meprobamate (Miltown)**. In the 1950s, Wallace laboratories, in an effort to maintain secrecy about their new drug, applied the code name **Miltown**, after the New Jersey borough. When the drug went to market in 1955, the company decided to keep the town name as the trade name.

Named originally for the peoples of the nation of Mongolia, the **Mongolian spot** is a melanocytic birthmark that may appear blue, or some shade of gray, black, or brown. The term was coined in 1883 by German anthropologist Erwin Bälz (1849–1913), who was actually working in Japan and not in Mongolia. In Mexico, the birthmark is called *rabo verde*, "green butt," and in Spanish the term sometimes used is *mancha* ("stain") *de Baelz* (Bälz), eponymously honoring the man who first described it. Mongolian spots generally disappear during later childhood.

The influenza pandemic of 1918–1920 is sometimes called the **Spanish flu**. Caused by the H1N1 virus, the disease affected 500 million people worldwide and resulted in more than 20 million deaths (Fig. 5.13). It seems ironic that Spain has

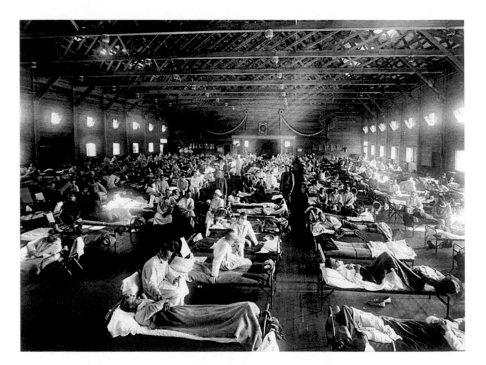

Fig. 5.13   The Spanish influenza. Emergency military hospital during influenza epidemic, Camp Funston, Kansas, USA. Source: *Pandemic Influenza: The Inside Story*. Nicholls H, PLoS Biology Vol. 4/2/2006, e50. Creative Commons. https://commons.wikimedia.org/wiki/File:Spanish_flu_hospital.png

had its name attached to a flu that has been traced to a single index case in a wholly different country: a US army cook at Fort Riley, Kansas.

Situated on the **hepatitis B virus (HBV)** is the surface antigen, a.k.a. the **Australia antigen (HBsAg)**. Its presence upon laboratory testing indicates current infection with the HBV. The name Australia antigen was suggested when American physician Baruch Blumberg (1925–2011) discovered its presence in the blood of a member of the Australian aboriginal population.

References

1. WHO issues best practices for naming new human infectious diseases. May 8, 2015. Available at: http://www.who.int/mediacentre/news/notes/2015/naming-new-diseases/en//
2. Piro A, et al. Casimir Funk: his discovery of the vitamins and their deficiency disorders. Ann Nutr Metab. 2010;57:85.
3. Jamieson HC. Catechism in medical history. Can Med Assn Jour. 1943;49:332.
4. Bollett AJ. Medical history in medical terminology. Res Staff Phys. 1999;45(9):60.
5. Atenstaedt RL. Trench fever: the British medical response in the Great War. J Roy Soc Med. 2006;99:564.
6. Taylor F, et al. The relation of peri-dental gingivitis to Vincent's angina. Proc Roy Soc Med. 1917;10:43.
7. McCormick C. Cape Cod a hot spot for babesiosis from ticks. Cape Cod Times. Available at: http://www.capecodtimes.com/article/20150418/NEWS/150419420

Chapter 6
Medical Metaphor, Simile, and Onomatopoeia

This chapter lumps together three somewhat similar types of medical words and phrases: **metaphor** and **simile**, things that seem like something else, and **echoic**, things that sound like something familiar to all. First let us examine metaphoric medical terms.

Greek philosopher Aristotle (384 BCE–322 BCE) considered the metaphor to represent the pinnacle of self-expression: "The greatest thing, by far, is to be a master of the metaphor. It is the one thing that cannot be learned and also is a sign of genius" [1]. Metaphor is an important part of medical discourse and is much more than a linguistic condiment. Where science strives for specificity, metaphor brings beguiling ambiguity, sometimes valuable to balance stark reality. For example, consider the metaphor that diabetes coats cells with sugar until they resemble tiny glazed donuts. On the other hand, metaphor can bring imagery to a complex concept. Sir Winston Churchill was subject to periodic spells of deep depression; he termed his depression "my black dog." There are medical metaphors that allude to weapons, sports, plants, trees, vegetables, fruits, seafood, cereals, crustaceans, and mythology.

American writer Anatole Broyard (1920–1990) observed, "Metaphors may be as necessary to illness as they are to literature, as comforting to the patient as his own bathrobe and slippers. At the very least, they are a relief from medical terminology. Perhaps only metaphor can express the bafflement, the panic combined with beatitude, of the threatened person" [2]. An example of the comfort that metaphor may bring to the patient, and perhaps also to the physician, lies in the Egyptian poem quoted by Periyakoil:

Death is before me today
Like the sky when it clears
Like a man's wish to see home after numberless years of captivity [3]

Canadian-American physician Sir William Osler (1849–1919) wrote the first comprehensive medical reference book and gave us many memorable quotations.

© Springer International Publishing AG 2017
R.B. Taylor, *The Amazing Language of Medicine*,
DOI 10.1007/978-3-319-50328-8_6

He gave us one of my favorite medical writing metaphors—a visual description of the aphorism as a "burr that sticks in memory" [4].

Physicians use metaphors in speaking with patients more than we might realize. In a 2010 study, Casarett et al. observed the interactions of 52 physicians with 94 patients with advanced cancer. They found that physicians used metaphors in two-thirds of all clinical conversations studied. Also, patient satisfaction was higher when the physician used metaphors [5].

Not only do physicians use metaphors, but our popular language has incorporated a number of "medical" metaphors in nonmedical contexts: the anemic growth of the stock market, injecting a dose of reality into the discussion, the timid person who lacks a spine, and a battle that reaches a fever pitch.

What about the simile? A favorite French saying is, "A meal without wine is like a day without sunshine." In 1794, Scottish poet Robert Burns (1759–1796) penned a song, "My Love is Like a Red, Red Rose." The simile, like the metaphor, creates an image by showing a clear comparison between two things. The simile is more explicit and generally involves more words than the metaphor. A metaphor, generally shorter, is more nuanced. "Her skin was like velvet" is a simile. "Her skin was velvet" is a metaphor.

Aristotle also had something to say about the simile: "The simile is a metaphor, differing from it only in the way it is put; and just because it is longer, it is less attractive" [1]. Thus the metaphor can be thought of as a compressed simile, with more vigor and inventiveness. You can often recognize a simile by the use of the word "like," as in "The lump in the woman's breast felt like a rock." And despite the opinion of Aristotle that the simile is "less attractive" than the metaphor, who cannot admire the recent conceptual image of a patient with advanced prostate cancer: "His bones were punched out like a train ticket at the end of the line, riddled with metastatic disease" [6]?

Onomatopoeia is like metaphor and simile in that it identifies something that is like something else. In the case of onomatopoeia, the "something" sounds like the noise made, for instance, when a bottle of carbonated beverage is opened (*fizz*) or the cry of a goose (*honk*). These "sound-like" words are also called echoic, from the mythological Echo, who adored Narcissus, cursed to be able only to repeat the last words uttered by others, as described in Chap. 2. Some echoic words familiar to everyone are hush, growl, clash, gulp, screech, moan, laugh, and chortle, the latter term created by British author Lewis Carroll (1832–1898), who also gave us *Alice's Adventures in Wonderland*. Another name for these words is imitative, as the names of many birds remind us of their calls: cuckoo, owl, bobwhite, and whippoorwill.

As intriguing as medical metaphors, similes, and echoic words may be, tracing them to their origins can be challenging. In many instances, they are the orphans, the parentless children, of our medical language. (Hint: Did you notice the metaphor in the previous sentence?) Few come directly from classic Greek and Latin, and many just seemed to evolve from everyday discourse. Nevertheless, they are part of medicine's core vocabulary, and there are a number of colorful stories, presented next.

Looks Like a Berry to Me

The **berry aneurysm** of the cerebral circulation is saccular in shape and may be tiny or as large as a few centimeters in diameter. As long as the aneurysm is intact, there are generally no symptoms. The danger is rupture, which can lead to subarachnoid hemorrhage, an intensely painful and life-threatening condition first fully described in 1924 by English neurologist Sir Charles P. Symonds (1890–1978). Seven years later, in 1931, British neurologist James Collier (1870–1935) identified and named what we now call the berry aneurysm [7]. The vascular abnormality was, indeed, named for its physical similarity to a small, juicy, round fruit, and there was no Doctor Berry involved. We value Dr. Collier's descriptive authorism as one example of a metaphor whose parentage is established in the literature.

Rice Water Stools

We associate **rice water stools** with **cholera**, a disease name that originated with the Greek word *kholera*, "a disease that causes diarrhea," with the suggestion that bile (*chole*) was somehow involved. This "causes diarrhea" descriptor would be a colossal understatement for the cholera manifestations we know today. And while we can trace the name of the disease, what about the metaphoric rice water stool?

Cholera seems to be a relatively new disease in the Western world. It was first described on the Indian subcontinent, notably the Ganges delta, with the early pandemics recorded in the nineteenth century. Sometimes called **Asiatic cholera**, it is a disease of poverty that occurs when drinking water is laced with sewage. A person with untreated cholera can lose up to 10–20 L of fluid to diarrhea in a day, and so-called cholera beds are cots with a hole strategically cut in the fabric (Fig. 6.1). Because of cholera's original association with Asia, and with rice as a staple of the diet among the area's inhabitants, it seems likely that the descriptor rice water stool originated there.

Some other colorful metaphors describing fecal contents in other settings include **pea soup stools** of typhoid, **anchovy sauce stools** of amoebic dysentery, **red currant jelly stools** of intussusception, and **tarry stools** of massive upper gastrointestinal bleeding.

Coffee, with Milk, Please

Sometimes a metaphor in a language other than English catches on, even if it requires a little knowledge of the non-English language to be understood. One of these is the *café au lait spot*, describing a flat pigmented macule (Fig. 6.2). Translated for those who never experienced high school French classes, *café au lait* means

Fig. 6.1 Cholera beds
made up with plastic sheets
and a hole for drainage.
Credit: Mark Knobil.
Creative Commons. https://
commons.wikimedia.org/
wiki/File:Cholera_
hospital_in_Dhaka.jpg

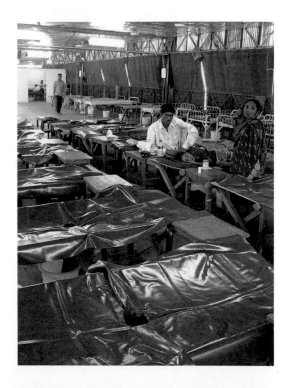

Fig. 6.2 A *café au lait*
spot on a patient's cheek,
with a US dime used to
indicate scale. Author:
T. Gnaevus Faber. Creative
Commons. https://
commons.wikimedia.org/
wiki/File:CALSpot.jpg

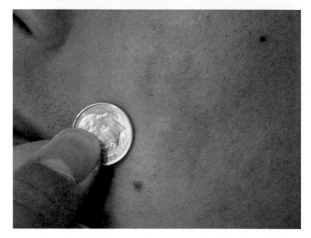

coffee with milk. Owing to their shape and sometimes variegated coloring, they are
also sometimes called **coast of Maine spots** or **giraffe spots**. Such macules are
likely to be harmless, but may be associated with neurofibromatosis type 1 or
McCune–Albright syndrome.

Physicians seem to have an affinity for culinary metaphors and the *café au lait*
spot is just one of many. Others include the **cheesy exudate** of thrush, **cauliflower**

ears that may follow trauma to the external ear, and **honey-colored crusts** of impetigo. The skin lesions of **pityriasis rosea** are often described as branny; then the word pityriasis comes from the Greek *pituron*, meaning "bran." For the Francophile, there is *peau d'orange* (**orange peel**) **skin** seen with cutaneous lymphatic edema.

On the Front Lines

There is an army of martial metaphors in medicine. In the early twentieth century, German scientist Paul Ehrlich (1854–1915) sought a **magic bullet** that would kill only the targeted organism, in this case the *Treponema* causing syphilis, as described further in Chap. 8.

Today we see **disease as the enemy**, we strive to augment the **body's defenses**, and we employ our **therapeutic armamentarium**. We **combat** heart disease, and we fight **invasive tumors** in our **war on cancer**. Describing his own struggle with metastatic prostate cancer, Irish historian Cornelius Ryan (1920–1974) writes:

> About the best I can say to you is that I feel as though a half-track has rolled back and forth across my stomach nonstop for several days. I have a neat tattoo of the entire beachhead right across my abdomen.... The attack was successful, although I am expecting a counter-attack any moment from all sides, if any more of those nodes are malignant. Notwithstanding, I have surrounded myself by barbed wire, land mines, and several squads of infantry, and we are ready to take on all comers. [8]

Of course, when the battle with a disease such as cancer becomes unwinnable, the combat imagery can make the transition to hospice care seem as though the war has been lost.

The Body as a Machine

Imbedded in the medical mentality, we often find the sense that the body is a machine, that disease is evidence that the machine is malfunctioning, and that the physician is the technician who can fix it. According to Periyakoil: "Machine metaphors are derived from Descartes' theory of mind and body duality by which the human body is seen as a machine with faulty parts that can removed and replaced. Going by this theory, all liver metastasis should be treatable with a liver transplant and all respiratory failures with ventilators" [3].

A commonly heard medical metaphor is the **train wreck**—a routine colonoscopy leads to a perforation, resulting in peritonitis, then sepsis, then pneumonia, and then a deep vein thrombosis, followed by a pulmonary embolism and perhaps even death. One problem crashes into the next organ. Incidentally, there also seems to be a strain of *sativa* (marijuana) called **train wreck** that hits the user like a freight train.

Other **machine metaphors** heard in the clinical setting are:

The patient is on **cruise control**.
We need to **fill up his tank**.
The agents help the body's immune apparatus **combat the tumor cells**.
We need to **fix your plumbing**.
Your **biological clock is ticking**.

Medicine as Sport

Lance Armstrong (born 1971) is a professional racing cyclist who won the Tour de France every year from 1999 to 2005. But before this amazing series of victories, he was diagnosed in 1996 with advanced testicular cancer, involving widespread metastases (Fig. 6.3). In his book *It's Not About the Bike: My Journey Back to Life*, Armstrong describes his bout with cancer through the eyes of an elite athlete:

> I had opened up a gap on the field. I knew that if I was going to be cured, that was the way it would go, with a big surging attack, just like in a race.... [the tumor markers HCG and AFP].... were my motivator, my yellow jersey.... I began to think of my recovery like a time trial in the Tour (de France).... I wanted to tear the legs off cancer, the way I tore the legs off other riders on a hill [9].

In patient care and in sport, we are part of a team—the **health-care team**, not "associates," as at Walmart. We explain to the patient that life has **thrown you a curve** and that we must **tackle the problem head-on**. We make a **game plan**, and **begin at the starting line**. We say that "Treatment is a marathon, and not a sprint," although I am not sure Lance Armstrong got this last message.

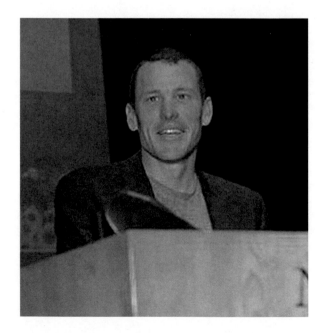

Fig. 6.3 Cyclist Lance Armstrong speaking at the National Institutes of Health. Source: NIH Record. Public Domain. https://commons. wikimedia.org/wiki/ File:NIH-lancearm2.jpg

Water Hammers, Phantom Limbs, and Thunderclap Headaches

The following is a potpourri of medical metaphors that don't fit categories such as sports, machinery, or military.

What is a **water hammer**? It is a child's toy, popular in the later nineteenth century, constructed of a cylinder half-filled with water, the balance of space being a vacuum. When the tube was inverted and then placed upright again, the impact of the water at each end would sound like a hammer hitting a nail. In 1832, Irish physician Sir Dominic Corrigan (1802–1880) described this phenomenon as characteristic of aortic regurgitation; it came to be known as the **Corrigan pulse**. Then in 1844, British physician Thomas Watson (1792–1882) made the metaphoric connection, and the term **water hammer pulse** was born. It is also sometimes called **Watson's water hammer pulse**.

As early as the sixteenth century, French surgeon Ambroise Paré (1510–1590) described the perception of pain and other sensations following amputation of a limb. Then in 1871, American physician and writer Silas Weir Mitchell (1829–1914) gave us the term **phantom limb**, found in more than half of all amputees. There is also a **phantom eye syndrome**—a sensation of eye pain and visual hallucinations after the removal of an eye. The word phantom comes from the Latin *phantasma*, meaning "an apparition."

The skin rash of **pityriasis rosea** gives us two colorful metaphors. The first is the **herald patch**, a large pigmented skin lesion that often occurs before the full-blown rash is evident. Following this initial manifestation, a number of oval-shaped, pink patches with a branny texture become evident on the chest, upper abdomen, and upper arms. These lesions sometimes occur in a **Christmas tree pattern** (Fig. 6.4). **Pityriasis rosea** has been misdiagnosed as a fungal infection of the skin or as secondary syphilis.

A headache that is intensely severe and that reaches maximum intensity quickly is called a **thunderclap headache**. In 1986, American neurologists Day and Raskin, at the University of California, San Francisco, gave us the term in a report of sudden headaches in a 42-year-old woman with a cerebral aneurysm [10].

An **orphan disease** is one that affects very few people. Most of these rare diseases are genetic. The most uncommon of all is ribose-5-phosphate isomerase deficiency, with only a single patient known to have the disease. An **orphan drug** is one developed to treat one of these rare diseases. The US Orphan Drug Act grants special status to these pharmaceutical products.

The **slapped cheek syndrome** is also called **erythema infectiosum** or **fifth disease** (Fig. 6.5); the latter term is from a list of causes of erythematous rashes compiled in the early 1900s (see Chap. 9). The disease causes bright red cheeks, as though the child has been slapped, along with a lacy rash that may cover most of the body.

Fig. 6.4 Christmas tree
distribution of the rash of
pityriasis rosea. Credit:
James Heilman,
MD. Creative Commons.
https://commons.
wikimedia.org/wiki/
File:Pityriasisrosa.png

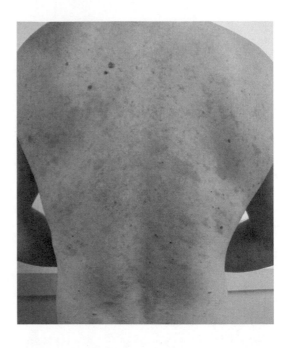

Fig. 6.5 A 14-month-old
boy with fifth disease.
Credit: Sandyjameslord.
Creative Commons. https://
commons.wikimedia.org/
wiki/File:14_month_old_
with_Fifth_Disease.jpg

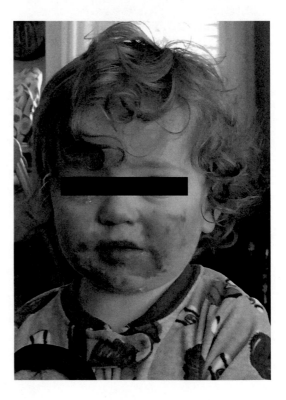

The **allergic salute** describes the habitual gesture of wiping mucus from the nose using the index finger or palm of the hand. Also sometimes called the **nasal salute**, it is seen in people with chronic allergic rhinitis.

The **swimmer's itch**, also sometimes called **duck itch**, **lake itch**, or **clam digger's itch**, is a pruritic dermatitis caused by larval forms of water-borne schistosomes. The parasites use freshwater snails as hosts, and wading or swimming in snail-infested freshwater streams or lakes can be hazardous. The itch is a short-term immune reaction to the organism, usually lasting only for a week or two.

There is a new favorite medical metaphor, the **parachute trial**, used to describe a study that examines a treatment that we all know to be effective or a fact we all know to be true. The metaphor alludes to the question of whether or not we need a research trial to validate that parachutes save lives of persons who jump from airplanes. A hypothetical example of a parachute trial would be a research study to determine if antibiotic therapy of community-acquired pneumonia is more effective than placebo. An actual example, in my opinion, is the study published in JAMA in 2016, with more than 60 coauthors, that concluded that "genetically elevated maternal BMI (body mass index) and blood glucose levels were potentially causally associated with higher offspring birth weight…" [11]. Translated: Overweight mothers from overweight families have overweight newborns. Funding of such studies is one more heartwarming example of our tax money at work.

Elephants, Serpents, and Fish

The **elephant disease**, also called **elephantiasis tropica** or **lymphatic filariasis**, is a chronic disease seen in tropical areas in which the patient's lymphatic channels become blocked by infection with mosquito-borne parasitic roundworms. In time the extremities, especially the legs and feet, come to resemble those of elephants (Fig. 6.6). The genitalia may be involved. Most common in Africa and Asia, more than 100 million persons worldwide are infected with the disease.

A **serpentine rash** characterizes cutaneous larva migrans. The intensely pruritic vesicular rash typically follows a wavy path and is commonly called **creeping eruption** or **ground itch**. The cause is a hookworm from the intestines of animals that penetrates exposed skin surfaces and can be contracted by walking barefoot on sandy beaches contaminated with animal feces. "Serpentine" refers to the twisting motion of a snake as it moves across the ground.

Ichthyosis describes a number of diseases manifested as extremely dry, scaly skin (Fig. 6.7). Most causes of ichthyosis are genetic. The disease name comes from the Greek *ichthys*, meaning "fish." In the past, people with ichthyosis sometimes were displayed in carnival sideshows as alligator boys or girls, along with the bearded lady and the dwarf. Dogs, as well as people, can have ichthyosis. American bulldogs, Jack Russell terriers, and golden retrievers are the breeds most at risk.

Fig. 6.6 Clinical portrait
(artotype) of elephantiasis
by the photographer O. G.
Mason; published in: Fox
GH. *Photographic
Illustrations of Skin
Diseases*. New York: EB
Treat; 1880. Public
Domain. https://commons.
wikimedia.org/wiki/
File:Elephanti.jpg

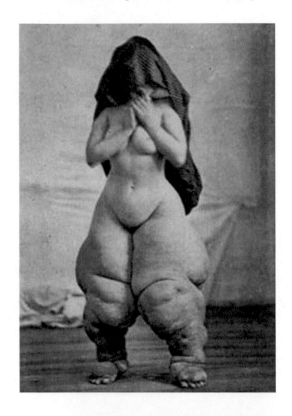

Fig. 6.7 Ichthyosis.
Source: Fox GH.
*Photographic Illustrations
of Skin Diseases, 2nd
edition*. New York: EB
Treat; 1886. Public
Domain. https://commons.
wikimedia.org/wiki/
File:Ichthyosis_1.jpg

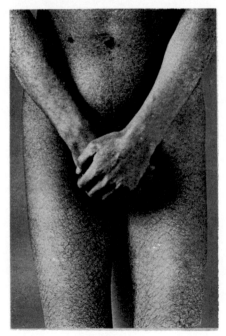

Things That Look Like Other Things

Many medical words come from the similarity of a body part or disease to some unrelated item. I think of these as implied metaphors or similes. Here are a few of them.

The **mitral valve** is a bicuspid valve located between the left atrium and left ventricle of the heart. It has two tapered leaves, and its appearance is similar to the shape of the tall hat worn by a bishop or cardinal—the mitre, a word that comes from Greek *mitra*, meaning "turban or belt" (Fig. 6.8).

A triangular membrane extending across the sclera, threatening to impair vision by covering the pupil, is called a **pterygium**. The abnormal tissue has a "winglike" appearance, and the name comes from the Greek *pterygion,* or "wing." Because the risk of developing a pterygium is increased with exposure to the sun's harmful ultraviolet rays, it is sometimes called **surfer's eye**.

The **placenta** is an organ connecting mammalian mothers and unborn infants during pregnancy. The word is directly taken from Latin, and in that language means "flat cake." Delivery of the **placenta**, after the emergence of the infant, is the "third stage of labor." What happens to the placenta subsequently may depend on where you live. The Māori of New Zealand and the Navajo peoples of the Southwestern United States bury the placenta. Native Hawaiians plant the placenta with a tree, believing that the "flat cake" is part of the infant and that the child and tree can grow together. In China, the placenta is sometimes used in traditional medications, and a few societies practice placentophagy—eating the human placenta (Fig. 6.9).

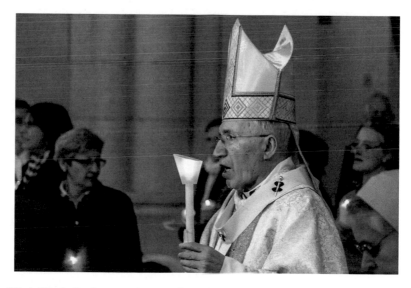

Fig. 6.8 A "bivalve" mitre worn by a cardinal of the Catholic Church in Madrid. Author: Barcex. Creative Commons. https://commons.wikimedia.org/wiki/File:Madrid_-_Catedral_de_la_Almudena_-_Rouco_Varela_-_130202_121510.jpg

Fig. 6.9 Human placenta shown a few minutes after birth. The side shown faces the baby with the umbilical cord top right. The unseen side connects to the uterine wall. The white fringe surrounding the bottom is the remnants of the amniotic sac. Photo by Jeremy Kemp. Public Domain. https://commons. wikimedia.org/wiki/ File:Human_placenta_ baby_side.jpg

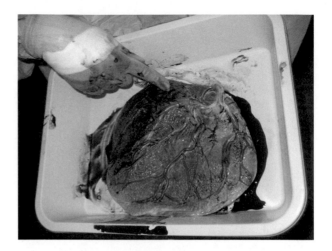

The disease **chicken pox**, properly called **varicella**, may have nothing to do with chickens; or it might. Dirckx (p. 26) tells that the term "is probably derived, a little irregularly, from Middle English *chiche*, 'chick-pea,' from Latin *cicer* of the same meaning." Haubrich, on the other hand, (p. 43) states, "Chicken pox is said to be so called not because the disease was thought to come from the familiar fowl but to distinguish its typically mild course from that of the more grave smallpox." As evidence, he cites other examples of the pettiness of anything related to our favorite source of eggs and drumsticks: "chicken-out," "chicken-hearted," and "chicken-feed." Chicken pox, although admittedly a usually minor disease, can become highly troublesome when reactivated later in life as **herpes zoster infection**.

That infection is perhaps more commonly known by the term **shingles**, which comes from the Latin *cingulum*, or "girdle," alluding to the tendency of the rash to encircle the body, if only to the midline. The Greek word *zoster* means "girdle." The word **herpes** comes from the Greek word *herpein*, meaning "to creep." English physician Richard Bright (1789–1858), remembered today for the eponymous Bright disease of the kidney, was the first to suggest that the disease was not a skin infection, but instead was based in the dorsal nerve root ganglia.

Our word **cancer** can be traced from Sanskrit (*karkatah*), to Greek (*karkinos*), to Latin (*cancer*). All mean "crab." The metaphor describes how malignant growths cling with crab-like tenacity to the tissues they invade. Greek physician Claudius Galen (129–200) likened cancer to the shape of a crab: "Just as a crab's feet extend from every part of the body, so in this disease (cancer) the veins are distended, forming a similar figure" (Haubrich, p. 36). An earlier meaning for the Sanskrit *karkatah* is "hard," and this root meaning has given us other words along with cancer. The first stage of syphilis is the **chancre**, which has a hard base. The word chancre shares its source with the word cancer, as does the familiar **canker sore** of the mouth.

Anthrax, the Greek word for "coal," describes the disease we know today. The metaphor suggests the skin lesions that are characterized by a coal-black eschar surrounded by fiery red inflammation—not unlike a burning ember (Fig. 6.10). The

Fig. 6.10 Cutaneous anthrax of the neck. Source: Centers for disease control and prevention's public health image library. Public Domain. https:// commons.wikimedia.org/ wiki/File:Cutaneous_ anthrax_lesion_on_the_ neck._PHIL_1934_lores. jpg

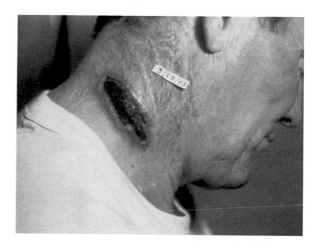

use of the word anthrax to describe the disease in the English language first appeared in a 1398 translation of *De Proprietatibus Rerum* (*On the Properties of Things*), a book by Parisian scholar Bartholomaeus Anglicus (1203–1272) that was originally published in 1240. Often associated with sheep and wool, anthrax is sometimes called **woolsorters' disease.** Another name for the disease is *la maladie de Bradford*; in its day, the English city of Bradford in West Yorkshire was called "the wool capital of the world." Anthrax lesions of the skin have also been called **hide porter's disease,** referring to the infection being contracted from infected animal hides.

Lupus means "wolf" in Latin. Tuberculosis of the skin is called **lupus vulgaris** and is manifested as painful cutaneous nodules. The "lupus" in this case refers to the destructive nature of the disease, as if being devoured by a wolf. **Lupus erythematosus,** an autoimmune disorder, is characterized by a butterfly-shaped malar rash that resembles a wolf's face. The "lupus" in lupus erythematosus may have arisen from the similarity of the butterfly rash to facial cutaneous tuberculosis—lupus vulgaris. Or it may have been a mistaken notion that the disease was caused by a wolf's bite [12].

Not all implied metaphors come from Greek, Latin, or modern English. One that has come to us from China is **ginseng,** from *renshen*, with *ren* meaning "man" and *shen* "an herb." The metaphor is that the ginseng plant resembles the shape of a man (Fig. 6.11). Ginseng has a special American connection: In his diary, US President George Washington (1732–1799) mentions the harvesting of the plant, and in the 1780s, American frontiersman Daniel Boone (1734–1820) was an active ginseng trader. Today ginseng enjoys considerable popularity. I recently researched current prices of ginseng online: Dried wild ginseng root aged 15–40 years and with a neck of two to three inches brings an amazing $800–$1400 or more per pound.

A disease name describing what one sees is **chikungunya,** caused by a mosquito-borne virus. Chikungunya means "that which bends up" in Makonde, a language spoken in southeast Tanzania and northern Mozambique. First discovered in Tanzania in 1952, the disease is now seen in other regions of Africa, Asia, and South

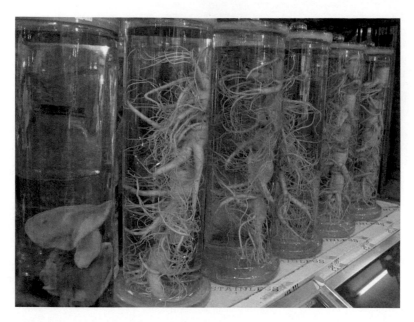

Fig. 6.11 Ginseng in a Korean market. Photographer: Richardfabi. Creative Commons. https://commons.wikimedia.org/wiki/File:Ginseng_in_Korea.jpg

America. Symptoms of chikungunya include fever accompanied by the severe joint and muscle pains that give rise to the manifestations behind the metaphoric "that which bends up."

The Shape of Things Medical

This section of the chapter could well be called the den of the –*oid* words. The suffix –*oid* is a Latin derivative of the Greek word *eidos*, meaning "form." I will begin with two words we all know: mastoid and thyroid.

The **mastoid process** of the temporal bone was named by Galen, who likened the conical prominence to a woman's breast, calling upon the word *mastos*, what the Greeks called the female mammary gland (Fig. 6.12). The mastoid process communicates with the middle ear and it contains many sinuses. In the good old days before antibiotics, a middle ear infection sometimes led to **mastoiditis**, requiring surgical drainage, an operation first performed by Paré in the sixteenth century. Originating on sternum and clavicle is the **sternocleidomastoid muscle**, with its insertion on the mastoid process.

Belgian anatomist Andreas Vesalius (1514–1564) first described what we now call the **thyroid gland** while working at the University of Padua in Italy. But the name **thyroid** is credited to English physician Tomás Wharton (1610–1673), who we remember for his discovery of the excretory duct of the submandibular gland,

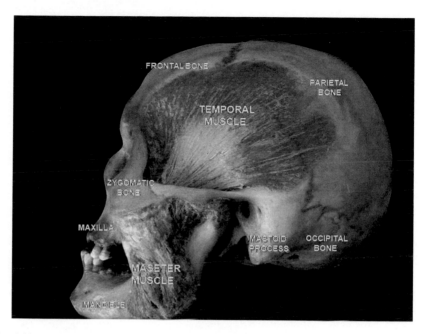

Fig. 6.12 Mastoid process. Source: Anatomist90. Creative Commons. https://commons.wikimedia.org/wiki/File:Slide1geo.JPG

now known as **Wharton's duct**. The name thyroid is taken from the Greek *thyreos*, describing the shield carried by warriors in Ancient Greece.

The suffix *–oid* is part of many other medical terms. Here are a dozen:

Medical term	Looks like—from Latin or Greek
Amyloid	Starch
Android	Resembling a man
Athetoid	Writhing
Cricoid	A ring
Deltoid	Delta, the triangular fourth letter of the Greek alphabet
Keloid	A crab's claw
Lipoid	Something fatty or greasy
Odontoid	A tooth
Osteoid	Bone
Scaphoid	A boat
Sigmoid	Sigma, eighteenth letter of the Greek alphabet
Xiphoid	A sword

Snap, Crackle, and Pop

Next I will present some **echoic** words, describing things that sound like something else. The names of cartoon characters associated since the 1940s with the Kellogg's cereal Rice Krispies—Snap, Crackle, and Pop—are, at least, partly imitative. The three words—names of the three imps pictured on the cereal box—are echoic of the sound created when milk is poured over the crisped rice shells. Such words are examples of **onomatopoeia**, coming from Greek *onoma* ("word or name") and *poiein* ("to compose"). Other echoic words used in everyday speech include: **buzz, hiss, beep, mumble,** and **whoosh. Swoosh,** the Nike footwear company trademark, is based on an echoic word. The word echoic has been co-opted by medical ultrasonography, resulting in its progeny—echogenic, hyperechoic, hypoechoic, and anechoic.

Some echoic terms enter the medical language as remodeling of Latin or Greek imitative words. One of these is *crepitus*, the Latin word for "rattle or crack." A fractured bone may exhibit **crepitus**—a grating sound—as the two fragments rub together; elicitation of crepitus in this situation is extremely painful and not generally advised. A crackling sound, **subcutaneous crepitus,** may be heard when there is air under the skin, as in the case of gas gangrene. Many older persons know the grinding crepitus caused by arthritis of the knees.

A similar echoic word is **fremitus,** a palpable or audible vibration somewhere in the body. Like crepitus, the word fremitus is taken directly from Latin, with the meaning "a growling." There is **pleural fremitus,** caused by a pleural friction rub. There is **bronchial fremitus,** caused by partial airway obstruction. And there is **tactile vocal fremitus,** felt by the examiner's hand as the patient repeats phrases like "blue balloon" or "toy boat." But never "ninety-nine," the use of which represents a long-propagated misunderstanding that began when some unnamed physician translated the number from the original German report in which the recommended low-frequency diphthong combination was *Neun und Neunzig.*

Cough

English writer Samuel Johnson (1709–1784) (Fig. 6.13) defined **cough** as: "A convulsion of the lungs, vellicated by some sharp serosity" (Forsyth, p. 143). There is no Latin or Greek source of the word cough. It entered the English language from the Dutch *kuchen*, and the Anglo-Saxon *cobbain*, both meaning "to cough," and the German *keuchen*. All these ancestral words are considered echoic. Reactive airway disease, gastroesophageal reflux disease, foreign body, angiotensin-converting enzyme inhibitors, "cough habit," and especially infection are all causes of cough. Infectious causes of cough include bronchitis, pneumonia, and tuberculosis, the latter highly feared in the nineteenth century (see Chap. 3). Another cause of cough is pertussis.

Fig. 6.13 A portrait of Samuel Johnson by Joshua Reynolds (1723–1792). Public Domain. https:// commons.wikimedia.org/ wiki/File:Samuel_ Johnson_by_Joshua_ Reynolds_2.png

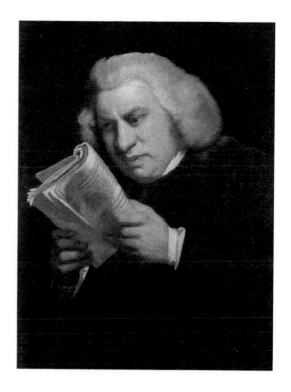

Maybe Not Exactly Like a Crane

Pertussis is the proper name of **whooping cough**, but the latter echoic term is firmly fixed in the popular lexicon. Sometimes the disease is called the **100-day cough**. The disease was once called hooping cough, until some time a few centuries ago, a "w" was added to give us whooping cough.

The term **pertussis** comes from the modern Latin prefix *per-*, meaning "thoroughly," attached to *tussis*, meaning "cough." Use of this term can be traced to British physician Thomas Sydenham (1624–1689), but was almost certainly used earlier.

I would like to tell that the term is imitative of the cry of the whooping crane, but can find no evidence for this theory. The "whooping" term comes from the Old French word *houper*, meaning "to cry out." The term whooping cough can foster a clinical misconception: The whoop is not the sound of the patient's expiratory cough, but instead is heard as the patient struggles to inspire after the paroxysm.

Sneezing and Sternutation

Our word **sneeze** comes from the Old English of the High Middle Ages, a language used around the year 1000. The word at that time was *fneosan*, to "sneeze or snort." This word, however, had precursors in Old High German and Old Norse. Over the ensuing centuries, the spelling evolved, notably with the addition of "s," and by the mid-seventeenth century, we find the first use of our current word **sneezing** in *Pseudodoxia Epidemica*, published in 1646 by English author Sir Thomas Browne (1605–1682):

> Concerning Sternutation or Sneezing, and the custom of saluting or blessing upon that motion, it is pretended and generally believed to derive its original from a disease wherein Sternutation proved fatal, and such as Sneezed died.... Yet Sneezing being properly a motion of the brain, suddenly expelling through the nostrils what is offensive to it, it cannot but afford some evidence of mental vigour [13].

Yes, **sternutation** is a perfectly good English word, describing the action of sneezing. And this brings me to the **ACHOO syndrome**.

In this book I have, so far, resisted the siren call of the acronym, an abbreviation formed from the first letters of words in a phrase, and used as a word itself, such as GERD (gastroesophageal reflux disease) and LASER (light amplification by stimulated emission of radiation). But the **ACHOO syndrome** is too tempting to resist. In 1987, Morris published a paper describing the **photic sneeze reflex**, the urge to sneeze upon exposure to bright light. Morris, as authors are wont to do, devised an acronym for the disorder: the ACHOO syndrome, standing for "autosomal-dominant compelling helio-ophthalmic outburst syndrome" [14]. I'll tell more about acronyms in Chap. 9.

There may be a word for the **ACHOO syndrome**. A **bacronym** is an acronymic word created first, and then the author constructs a phrase with words containing first letters to fit the letters in the word created. An example is the familiar **AMBER alert**, officially an acronym for "America's Missing: Broadcast Emergency Response," but actually the name of a Texas girl named Amber whose abduction and murder in 1996 inspired creation of the program.

Spit and Sputum

The common word **spit**, imitative of the sound made during expectoration, comes from Anglo-Saxon *spitu* and *spittan*. The word refers to the forceful evacuation of a fluid, classically saliva, a favorite activity of those who use chewing tobacco. In my youth, our town barbershop had a handy spittoon (Fig. 6.14). In ancient times, spittle was thought to have curative properties. The concept appears in the biblical verse Mark 8:23:

> And he took the blind man by the hand, and led him out of the town; and when he had spit on his eyes, and put his hands upon him, Jesus asked him if he saw ought. And he looked up, and said, I see men as trees, walking.

The word **sputum** comes from Latin *spuere*, meaning "to spit." This descriptor of mixed saliva and respiratory tract mucus is also considered to be of echoic origin. Each year pulmonologists and respiratory therapists gather for the American Association for Respiratory Care's national convention. A highlight of this continu-

Fig. 6.14 Line art drawing of a spittoon. Source: Pearson Scott Foresman. Public Domain. https://commons.wikimedia.org/wiki/File:Spittoon_(PSF).png

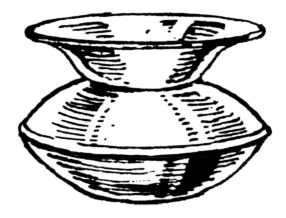

ing medical education meeting is the **Sputum Bowl**, a test of knowledge using a format similar to the television quiz show *Jeopardy*, with teams, buzzers, and intense competition for bragging rights.

Hiccup or Hiccough?

An uncontrollable diaphragmatic spasm punctuated by a sudden closure of the glottis is a **hiccup**, a term that when pronounced sounds remarkably like what it describes. Some, more refined souls, have used the word **hiccough**, linguistically incorrect simply because the phenomenon is not a cough. Obsolete synonyms are **hickop** and **hicket**, definitely superior to hiccough, but now in the etymologic wastebasket (Evans and Evans, p. 220).

The all-time record holder for hiccups, according to the venerable *Guinness Book of World Records*, is American Charles Osborne, who suffered hiccups for 68 years, resulting in an estimated 430 million diaphragmatic spasms.

Murmur, Innocent and Otherwise

When heard through the stethoscope, the **murmur** is a sound produced by turbulence as blood crosses a heart valve. The word comes directly from Latin, where it means "hum, muttering, or rushing," a translation that seems a lot like murmurs as we know them today. Not every **murmur** indicates disease, and many are "physiologic," "functional," or "innocent."

The use of the stethoscope to distinguish harmless from ominous murmurs is a time-honored component of the diagnostic examination. But that method is now challenged by the portable ultrasound, and medical students sometimes acquire these devices early in their training. Today the question is being asked, "Will the ultrasound replace the stethoscope?" Gillman et al. have stated: "Using ultrasound not as a diagnostic test, but instead as a component of the physical exam, may allow it to become the stethoscope of the twenty-first century" [15]. Will young physicians of the future lose the ability to recognize the holosystolic murmur of mitral regurgitation or the opening snap of mitral stenosis? Will the stethoscope be relegated to a fashion accessory draped around the neck? Is René Laennec spinning in his grave?

Rumble in the Jungle

Borborygmus is, to use a metaphoric definition, elephantine rumbling of the bowels. The word has respectable classic ancestors, Latin *borborigmus*, and earlier *borborygmos*, from Ancient Greek, both describing audible gas movement in the intestine. Although its birth record is lost in history, the word is almost certainly of onomatopoetic origin. Sometimes described as growling or gurgling, the sounds can sometimes be heard across the room.

Health professionals do not have exclusive rights to the word borborygmus, which has been used to describe various noise-producing systems, including plumbing. In his 1969 novel *Ada*, Russian-American novelist Vladimir Nabokov (1899–1977), who also gave us *Lolita*, wrote: "All the toilets and water pipes in the house had been suddenly seized with borborygmic convulsions."

Piss and Pee and the Pequod That Wasn't

Yes, we physicians say **urine**, or **urinate**, but we cannot dismiss **piss** from medical history. The word comes from the Latin *pissiare*, of echoic origin. From there in the twelfth century in Old French we find *pissier*, meaning "urinate." In the sixteenth century, we had the **piss prophet**, a.k.a. the **water-scriger**, who diagnosed patients' ailments based on the appearance, odor, and taste of the urine. Thinking about it, the latter would be a reasonable way to diagnose diabetes. The public urinal in France (and some other European countries) is the *pissoir* (Fig. 6.15).

In the eighteenth century, **pee** meant "to spray with urine," and today seems to be a euphemism, based on the initial letter of piss, that is most often heard in discourse with children. Piss and pee are used as both nouns and verbs.

The word pee is the key part of an etymologic tale, a story of a naming that never happened (Forsyth, p. 179). In Seattle, Washington, a young English teacher and two friends planned to start an upscale coffee shop. The English teacher, Jerry Baldwin, loved Herman Melville's 1851 allegory of a man and a huge white whale, *Moby Dick*. Baldwin proposed a name for the new coffee shop—Pequod, the name of Captain Ahab's ship. His partners questioned the wisdom of naming a shop sell-

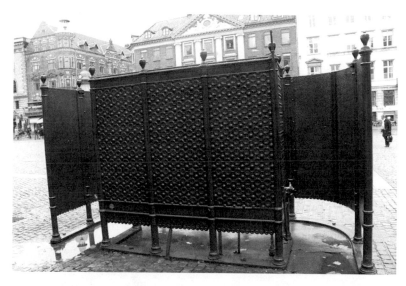

Fig. 6.15 Pissoir (urinal) in cast-iron from Copenhagen. Author: Bjørn som tegner. Creative Commons. https://commons.wikimedia.org/wiki/File:Pissoir_1.JPG

ing fluids with as word that sounded like pee. So it was back to the book. The final choice: **Starbucks**, derived from the name of the Pequod's first mate.

In 2016, the *New York Daily News* featured a story titled "Drink Your Own Urine in Cocktail Form," telling how to make pee-laced mixed drinks such as "Long Island Iced Pee," "Piss-co Sour," and "Octapissy." It turns out that, in the words of the author, "They're a gag—in every sense" [16].

Quacks and Quacksalvers

An unqualified, and often unscrupulous, person claiming special healing powers is called a **quack**. Often the quack has a panacean elixir to sell (Fig. 6.16). The term can be traced to the Middle Ages, the time of the plague. This onomatopoetic term comes from Dutch *quacksalver*, describing one who quacks like a duck as he hawks his marvelous remedies (Ciardi, p. 320). *Quacksalver*, in turn, came from the Middle Dutch words *quacken*, "to boast," and *salven*, "to rub with ointment."

Is quackery a historical curiosity? No, not even in the twenty-first century. Using a Delphi method, Norcross et al. studied 59 psychological treatments and tests in current use to determine which had been discredited. Of these, 14 were found to be "certainly discredited." These included crystal healing, past lives therapy, orgone therapy, rebirthing therapy, and aromatherapy [17]. And let's not forget iridology, Pacific Ocean shark cartilage, and psychic surgery. Yes, quackery is alive and well in the twenty-first century.

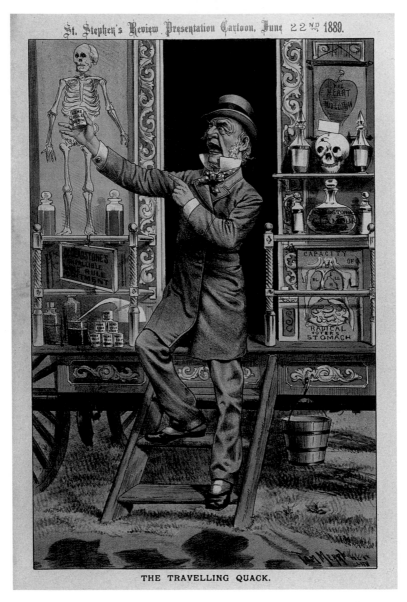

Fig. 6.16 A quack doctor selling remedies from his caravan. Source: Chromolithograph by T. Merry, 1889. Public Domain. https://commons.wikimedia.org/wiki/File:A_quack_doctor_selling_remedies_from_his_caravan;_satirizing_Wellcome_V0011377.jpg

References

1. Aristotle: Rhetoric: the complete works of Aristotle. Edited by Barnes J. Princeton: Princeton University; 1985, p. 2251.
2. Broyard A: Intoxicated by my illness and other writings on life and death. New York: Ballantine Books, 1992.

3. Periyakoil VS. Using metaphors in medicine. J Pall Med. 2008;11:842.
4. Taylor RB. On the shoulders of medicine's giants. New York: Springer; 2014, p. 62.
5. Casarett D, et al. Can metaphors and analogies improve communication with seriously ill patients? J Palliat Med. 2010;13:255.
6. Thurston A. The unreasonable patient. JAMA. 2016;315:657.
7. Collier J. Cerebral hemorrhage due to causes other than arteriosclerosis. Br Med J. 1931;2(3689):519.
8. Ryan C, Ryan KM: A private battle. London, United Kingdom, New English Library, 1981.
9. Armstrong L: It's not about the bike: my journey back to life. New York, NY: Putnam; 2000.
10. Day JW, Raskin NH. Thunderclap headache: symptom of unruptured cerebral aneurysm. Lancet. 1986;2(8518):1247.
11. Tyrrell J, et al. Genetic evidence for causal relationships between maternal obesity-related traits and birth weight. JAMA. 2016;315:1129.
12. Blotzer JW. Systemic lupus erythematosus: historical aspects. Maryland State Med J. 1983;32:439.
13. Browne T. Pseudodoxia epidemica. London: 1646.
14. Morris HH. ACHOO syndrome prevalence and inheritance. Cleve Clin Med. 1987;54:431.
15. Gillman LM. Portable bedside ultrasound: the visual stethoscope of the 21st century. Scand Trauma, Resusc, and Emerg Med. 2012, 20:18.
16. Cutler J. Drink your own urine in cocktail form. New York Daily News, Feb. 2, 2016. Available at: http://www.nydailynews.com/life-style/health/drink-urine-cocktail-form-article-1.2517558#
17. Norcross JC, et al. Discredited psychological treatments and tests: A Delphi poll. Prof Psychology: Res Pract. 2006;37:515.

Chapter 7
Eponymous and Honorary Medical Terms

When a disease is named after an author, it is very likely that we don't know much about it.
German surgeon August Bier (1861–1949) (Strauss, p. 116)

The quotation above by August Bier, the surgeon who performed the first operation under spinal anesthesia, seems to reflect—with good humor—an opinion in the ongoing controversy regarding eponyms. His skepticism notwithstanding, we honor Bier's memory with the eponymous **Bier block**, another name for intravenous regional anesthesia. But, of course, a procedure isn't a disease.

An eponym is a name derived from a noun, generally the name of a person. An example is the **Baker cyst** of the knee, named for English surgeon William Morrant Baker (1839–1896). In an interesting linguistic twist, the term eponym can also refer to the person for which something is named. That is, in this example, Baker can be considered the eponym for the popliteal cyst he described.

Diseases, procedures, tests, or anatomical parts named for someone have long been part of the medical landscape. Which physicians and scientists have had the most entities linked to their names? According to an undoubtedly reliable website describing a review of more than 900 pages of eponyms [1], these are the top five winners in the eponymic sweepstakes:

- The grand champion is French neurologist Jean Martin Charcot (1825–1893), honored with 20 medical eponyms. He is considered by many to be the "founder of modern neurology." His name has top billing in multi-eponymous **Charcot–Marie–Tooth disease**, a hereditary motor and sensory neuropathy. There are, in fact, two different **Charcot triads**, one a trio of clinical signs of multiple sclerosis and the other describing three common manifestations of ascending cholangitis.
- In second place is English surgeon and pathologist Sir James Paget (1814–1899). Among his 13 medical eponyms are **Paget disease of bone** and **Paget disease of the nipple**, the latter describing intraductal breast cancer that has spread to the skin around the nipple.

© Springer International Publishing AG 2017
R.B. Taylor, *The Amazing Language of Medicine*,
DOI 10.1007/978-3-319-50328-8_7

- We recall English surgeon Sir Percivall Pott (1714–1788) for his description of spinal tuberculosis, **Pott disease**, as well as a lower extremity fracture named for him—described later in this chapter—and several other entities, for a total of 11 eponyms.
- Next on the list is English surgeon and ophthalmologist Sir Jonathan Hutchinson (1828–1913), who has 10 eponyms to his name. The best known today is the **Hutchinson pupil**, a clinical finding in which the pupil is dilated and unreactive to light, seen on the side of an intracranial mass lesion.
- Tied with Hutchinson is German physician and pathologist Rudolf Virchow (1821–1902), considered "the father of modern pathology." He also has 10 medical eponyms, including the **Virchow node**, an enlarged, hard lymph node in the left supraclavicular space, suggesting the presence of a gastrointestinal cancer.

I was a little surprised that Hippocrates, Thomas Sydenham, and Sir Thomas Osler did not make the "top five," but data are data.

I mentioned above in the first paragraph that there are controversies surrounding the use of eponyms. One seemingly trivial spat has to do with possessives. Do we speak of Hutchinson's pupil or the Hutchinson pupil? The tendency in medical dictionaries is to drop the possessive, although no one seems to have noticed that by doing so, proper syntax now often calls for the article "the." We can have **Hutchinson's pupil** or **THE Hutchinson pupil**; choose one. In this book, I have made a bet on the eventual elimination of possessives and have presented eponyms minus the possessive case. An exception is when the disease was experienced by the patient for whom it is named, such as Lou Gehrig's disease.

But there other reasons eponyms are under attack today. One is duplication, with two different Charcot triads mentioned above and two quite different Addisonian diseases. There are no less than three Ramsay Hunt syndromes, linked only by each being first described by American neurologist James Ramsay Hunt (1872–1937).

Sometimes the eponym honors the wrong person, not the first to discover or describe something. The disease we know as **Wegener granulomatosis**, formally known as **granulomatosis with polyangiitis**, was described by Heinz Kinger and others before Wegener. Wegener's report came later, but the disease bears his name [2]. Or the eponym is chosen to honor someone who had nothing to do with the disease or discovery; for example, *Serratia*, a genus of Gram-negative bacteria, is named in honor of Italian physicist Serafino Serrati, who is credited (by Italians, at least) with the invention of the steamboat (Dirckx, p. 78).

Others point out that the use of an eponym can be different in different counties. For example, the disease **sideropenic dysphagia** is called **Waldenström–Kjellberg syndrome** in Scandinavia and **Paterson–Brown–Kelly syndrome** in the United Kingdom, while US physicians know it as **Plummer–Vinson syndrome**. **Graves disease** is named for Irish physician Robert James Graves, but depending on one's country, toxic diffuse goiter may also be called **Parry disease**, after English physician Caleb Hillier Parry (United Kingdom), or **Flajani disease**, after Italian physician Giuseppe Flajani (Italy).

The microbiologists seem to be quite fond of eponyms and honor their heroes such as German bacteriologist **Albert Neisser** (*Neisseria* **genus**), French scientist **Jules Bordet** (*Bordetella* **genus**), and Swiss bacteriologist **Alexandre Yersin** (*Yersinia* **genus**). They can also be fickle: *Yersinia pestis*, the bacterial cause of bubonic plague, was once *Pasteurella pestis*.

Some Philistines call for the abolition of all eponyms. In their paper titled "Should eponyms be abandoned? Yes," Woywodt and Matteson state: "Eponyms often provide a less than truthful account of how diseases were discovered and reflect influence, politics, language, habit, or even sheer luck rather than scientific achievement." They also discuss the few tainted eponyms, a topic I will discuss at the end of this chapter [2].

I, on the other hand, am an unapologetic eponymophile. To discard all our historical eponyms would jettison much of medicine's rich history and would leave us with many instances of barely intelligible descriptive nomenclature. Ask yourself: Would you rather consider Guillain–Barré syndrome or acute inflammatory demyclinating polyradiculoneuropathy? Isn't it easier to say Scheuermann disease than idiopathic juvenile kyphosis of the spine? Aren't two words better than six? Or how about Tay–Sachs disease versus GM2 gangliosidosis? In fact, entities such as Bartter syndrome, Marfan syndrome, Ménière disease, Waardenburg syndrome, and Whipple disease offer such complexity that descriptive nomenclature might consume half a paragraph.

And so, now that I have revealed my bias, let us explore the history of some of medicine's favorite eponyms.

Fingers, Facies, and Wreaths

As we launch into individual eponyms, it seems appropriate to begin with the "Father of Western Medicine," Hippocrates (460–370 BCE). **Hippocratic fingers**, also called **Hippocratic nails** or **digital clubbing**, describes an enlargement of the distal phalanges of the fingers, most often seen with diseases of the lungs or heart causing chronic hypoxia. Up to half of persons with non-small cell lung cancer will develop Hippocratic fingers.

One way to assess this involves **Schamroth's test**, named for South African cardiologist Leo Schamroth (1924–1988). In this test, the same fingers of the opposite hand are placed back-to-back and nail-to-nail. In normal persons a diamond-shaped window is seen between the nails. When clubbing is present, the window is absent. Schamroth, who had Hippocratic nails himself, is one of the patients for whom a disease or sign is named; some others are described later in the chapter.

In addition to Hippocratic nails, there is the **Hippocratic face**, or **facies** for the classical scholars among us, the facial evidence of cachexia that often precedes death due to chronic, progressive disease. In words that might have been those of Hippocrates:

Fig. 7.1 Image of
Hippocrates; note the
"Hippocratic wreath" of
male pattern baldness.
Source: Young Persons'
Cyclopedia of Persons and
Places, 1881. Public
Domain. https://commons.
wikimedia.org/wiki/
File:Hippocrates.jpg

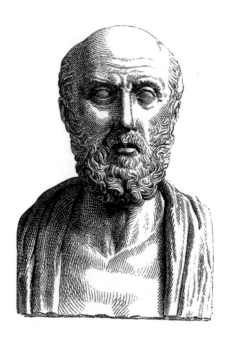

[If the patient's facial] appearance may be described thus: the nose sharp, the eyes sunken, the temples fallen in, the ears cold and drawn in and their lobes distorted, the skin of the face hard, stretched and dry, and the colour of the face pale or dusky . . . and if there is no improvement within [a prescribed period of time], it must be realized that this sign portends death. [3]

On a lighter note, there is also the **Hippocratic wreath**, describing the rim of hair at the rear and sides of the scalp seen with **male pattern baldness**, or **androgenic alopecia**, and just further evidence that bald men are smarter (Fig. 7.1).

The Circle and the Nerve of Willis

English neuroanatomist Thomas Willis (1621–1675) described the ring of blood vessels at the base of the brain that we now call the **circle of Willis** (Fig. 7.2) He also wrote of the cerebral neuroanatomy and the cranial nerves, including the **spinal accessory nerve**, sometimes called the **Willis nerve**.

The son of a farmer, Willis, like many young physicians, had an early clinical outcome that helped to enhance his reputation and bring patients to his practice. As described by Hughes, at age 29, Willis seemed to raise the dead. A 23-year-old woman, accused of murdering her child, was hanged. Her body was placed in a coffin and taken to Willis for autopsy. Willis opened the coffin to find the woman to be alive, and his fame for this apparent medical miracle spread rapidly. The woman, for her part, was pardoned and went on to marry and become mother of three more children [4].

Fig. 7.2 An MRI image of the circle of Willis. Source: Ceccomaster. Creative Commons. https://commons.wikimedia.org/wiki/File:Circle_of_Willis_-_MRI,_MIP_-_Anterior_projection.png

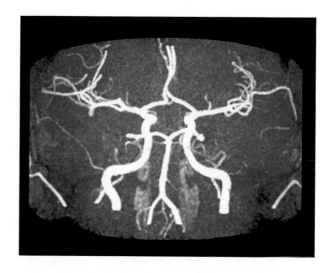

Willis contributed much to medicine, including coining the word *neurologie*, now **neurology**, a term that first appeared in his book *Cerebri Anatome* (The Anatomy of the Brain), published in 1664.

Colles Fracture and His Folly

All physicians are familiar with the distal radial fracture described in 1814 by Irish professor of surgery Abraham Colles (1773–1843) in his paper titled *On the Fracture of the Carpal Extremity of the Radius*. Because the distal radius fracture described by Colles is accompanied by dorsal and radial displacement of the wrist and hand, it is sometimes called a **dinner fork deformity**, but we are more likely to call it a **Colles fracture** (Fig. 7.3). (Note that Colles, like Graves, ends in "s" and there is no possessive in the eponym.)

Colles gave us even more eponyms: He studied the **inguinal ligament**, also called the **Colles ligament**, and the membranous layer of the subcutaneous tissue of the perineum, or **Colles fascia**. I can happily report, however, that few remember **Colles law**, described next.

Colles was a student of syphilis, a not uncommon disease in his day. He observed that a child born with congenital syphilis did not cause a lesion to form on the mother's breast while nursing, but could infect others who might nurse the infant. Colles concluded, incorrectly, that the mother was immune to the disease, and this dictum became **Colles law**. What Colles didn't recognize was that the mother already had the disease and thus would not manifest new signs of primary syphilis. **Colles law** prevailed for seven decades until challenged by German bacteriologist August Paul von Wassermann (1866–1925), recalled today as the man who, in 1906, developed the **Wassermann test for syphilis**.

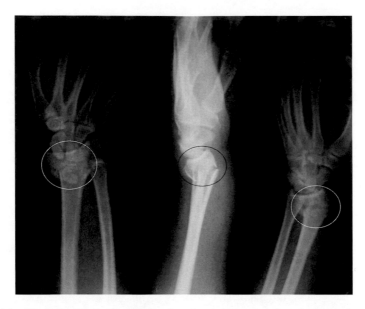

Fig. 7.3 An X-ray image of a fractured radius showing the characteristic Colles fracture with displacement and angulation of the distal end of the radius. Source: Ashish j29. Creative Commons. https://commons.wikimedia.org/wiki/File:Colles_fracture.JPG

Parkinson Disease

Scottish surgeon John Hunter (1728–1793) had a number of illustrious pupils. Among these were English country doctor Edward Jenner (1749–1823), who championed the use of **cowpox** as a vaccine against **smallpox**; English surgeon John Abernathy (1764–1831), who gave us the **Abernathy biscuit** as an aid to digestion; and English anatomist Astley Paston Cooper (1768–1841), known today for **Cooper's ligament** and other hernia-related miscellanea. Another of these students was James Parkinson.

If for nothing else, London physician James Parkinson (1755–1824) would be remembered for reporting, in 1812, the first case of appendicitis in the English language, also noteworthy in that the case described was the first instance in which perforation was recognized as the cause of death (Garrison, p. 424). But this primacy of reporting is overshadowed by his classic description of **paralysis agitans**, sometimes called the **hypokinetic rigid syndrome**.

Parkinson's 1817 monograph, titled *An Essay on the Shaking Palsy*, reported six persons with the disease. It included descriptions of the key disease manifestations: the characteristic resting tremor, the telltale posture, the shuffling gait, and weakened muscle strength. A half-century later, Jean-Martin Charcot (our etymology champion with 20 terms that bear his name, as described above) added to Parkinson's findings and led the effort to rename the disease to honor the man who gave us the classic description. Today we call it **Parkinson disease**, or even simply **parkinsonism**.

Story of a Flawed Giant

British physician Thomas Addison (1793–1860) has been the source of a number of medical eponyms. Best known is **Addison disease**, which he first described in his 1855 paper *On the Constitutional and Local Effects of Disease of the Suprarenal Capsules* [5]. Addison disease, or **primary adrenal insufficiency**, is a failure of the adrenal glands to produce needed steroid hormones. Addison's report described six cases, all caused by tuberculosis of the "suprarenal capsules," as the adrenal glands were once called.

There are other Addison eponyms. In connection with primary adrenal insufficiency, a severe and life-threatening failure of adrenal function is an **Addisonian crisis**. There is also **Addisonian anemia**, or **pernicious anemia**, caused by a failure to absorb vitamin B12. Then there is **Addisonism**, describing manifestations similar to Addison disease, such as bronze pigmentation of the skin, but not caused by loss of adrenocortical function.

Addison, one of medicine's giants, suffered depression, called **melancholia** (from the Greek words meaning "black bile") in his time. On June 29, 1860, Addison threw himself over a wall, fractured his frontal bone, and died.

About Spoiled Wine and a Boston Street

Louis Pasteur (1822–1895) was a French industrial chemist working to combat the spoilage of wine, the process whereby a fine adult beverage turns to vinegar (Fig. 7.4). Pasteur defined ferment as "a living form which originates from a germ" (Garrison, p. 576). In 1864, Pasteur discovered that heating wine to 55–60 degrees centigrade before corkage eliminated pathogens and reduced the number of germs enough to retard spoilage, without sacrificing bouquet or flavor (Bordley, p. 194). He patented the process the following year. His discovery was a great boon to the French wine industry, and the discovery that the same process—**pasteurization**—could render milk safe to drink has saved the lives of millions of infants.

Pasteur also did groundbreaking work on the concept of immunity in regard to chicken cholera and anthrax in cattle, aware that in 1796 Edward Jenner had shown that cowpox can produce immunity to smallpox. In preparing his agents of immunization, Pasteur called them **vaccines** to honor Jenner, even though, unlike cowpox, cows were not the source of his agents. Then in 1885, Pasteur and his colleagues developed a rabies **vaccine**, which they tested on nine-year-old Joseph Meister, who had been badly bitten by a rabid dog. For his part in this experimental use of a new vaccine, Pasteur, who was not a physician, put himself at legal risk. But the boy survived, and Pasteur evaded legal problems.

There is a Pasteur Institute in Paris, a UNESCO/Institute Pasteur Medal awarded biannually "in recognition of outstanding research contributing to a beneficial impact on human health," and there is an Avenue Louis Pasteur in Boston,

Fig. 7.4 Portrait of Louis
Pasteur, by Albert Edelfelt,
1885. Source: Paintingiant.
com. Public Domain.
https://commons.
wikimedia.org/wiki/
File:Tableau_Louis_
Pasteur.jpg

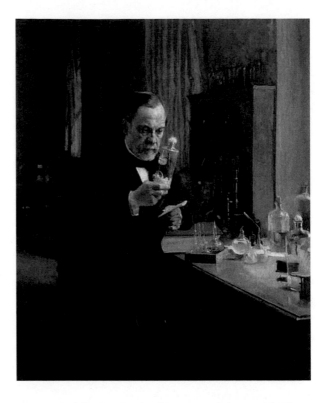

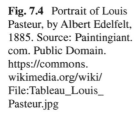

Fig. 7.4 Portrait of Louis Pasteur, by Albert Edelfelt, 1885. Source: Paintingiant.com. Public Domain. https://commons.wikimedia.org/wiki/File:Tableau_Louis_Pasteur.jpg

Massachusetts, and other streets named for Pasteur in cities around the world. There is the **Pasteur effect**: The process of fermentation is inhibited when oxygen is abundant. The **Pasteur pipette** is a tapered glass laboratory pipette. And there is the **Pasteurella genus** of bacteria, in the family ***Pasteurellaceae***. Louis Pasteur has been thoroughly and properly "eponymized."

The Unwelcome Naming

Building on the discoveries of Pasteur, British surgeon Joseph Lister (1827–1912) is remembered as the innovator of antiseptic surgery. He found that liberal use of **carbolic acid**, now called **phenol**, during surgery reduced the incidence of infections. Why did Lister choose this particular chemical for his 1867 experiment? Lister had noticed that when carbolic acid was used to quell the stench of sewage waste used to irrigate fields near the city of Carlisle, England, it produced no ill effects in animals later grazing in the area. So why would it not be an effective antiseptic and yet equally benign in humans during surgery?

In addition to spraying surgical incisions, instruments, and dressings with carbolic acid, Lister insisted that surgeons wash their hands with a carbolic acid solution and wear clean gloves for each procedure. In 1876, Lister described his antiseptic surgical technique at the International Medical Congress in Philadelphia. Despite some initial skepticism, the method, called **listerism**, caught on in America and around the world, helping to give us the (usually) safe surgery we enjoy today.

In 1879, American chemist Joseph Lawrence marketed an antiseptic mouthwash, which Lawrence named **Listerine**, either to honor Lister or to traffic on his fame, perhaps both. Lawrence teamed up with an American pharmacist named Jordan Wheat Lambert, who marketed Listerine through his new company, Lambert Pharmacal Company of St. Louis, Missouri.

Listerine was promoted to dentists for use as a mouthwash that could cure bad breath. As early as 1921, there was also **Listerine toothpaste** (Fig. 7.5). Over the years, Listerine was also touted to be useful for colds, sore throat, and dandruff. It was briefly claimed to be a cure for gonorrhea. In 1927, Lambert Pharmaceuticals marketed **Listerine cigarettes**.

What actually is in Listerine? It is a combination of menthol, eucalyptol, thymol, and methyl salicylate—all in a solution that is 21 % alcohol. (For those who are not familiar with distilled spirits, most vodka and whiskey sold today is 40 % alcohol, expressed as "80 proof.") There is no carbolic acid/phenol at all in Listerine.

All of this was without Lister's approval, and he was not amused. In fact, according to Dirckx (p. 82), Lister spent considerable energy and personal funds in a battle against the mouthwash and the company that had placed his name on a product that was unrelated to his work. Despite Lister's efforts, Listerine caught on, and Lambert Pharmaceuticals went on to become Warner-Lambert Pharmaceuticals, subsequently acquired by Pfizer in 2000. The surgeon may have disavowed the mouthwash, but some of his descendants still receive royalties from sales of Listerine (Li, p 46).

There are actually enduring scientific eponyms for Lister. *Listerella* is a genus of slime mold, and *Listeria* is genus of bacteria, notable in humans for *Listeria monocytogenes*, the cause of the food-borne infection **listeriosis**.

Robert Koch and His Postulates

The accomplishments of German physician and microbiologist Robert Heinrich Hermann Koch (1843–1910) have prompted a number of eponyms. He discovered the etiologic agent of tuberculosis (TB), and, for this achievement, he was awarded the 1905 Nobel Prize in Physiology or Medicine. The organism causing TB has been called the **Koch bacillus**. Koch discovered the bacterial cause of anthrax, and also *Haemophilus aegyptius*, sometimes called the **Koch-Weeks bacillus**—the cause of an infectious form of human conjunctivitis.

There is also the **Koch phenomenon**, another name for the delayed hypersensitivity response, and **Koch sterilization**, a method of disinfection using steam. But what we most recall is the logical construct called **Koch's postulates**.

A postulate is an analytical judgment that we use as a principle. Here's an example. In mathematics we postulate that things equal to the same things are equal to

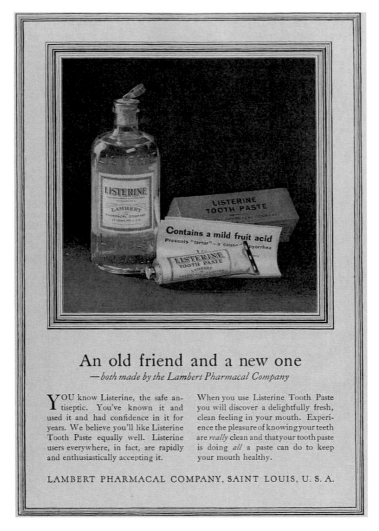

Fig. 7.5 Listerine advertisement in the June 1921 *Photoplay* magazine. Public Domain. https://commons.wikimedia.org/wiki/File:Listerine_Ad_-_June_1921_Photoplay.jpg

each other. Thus: Two plus three equals five; one plus four equals five; therefore two plus three equals one plus four.

Since 1890, Koch's postulates hold that we can say that a given organism is the cause of a given disease only if the following conditions are met:

- The bacteria must be present in every case of the disease.
- The bacteria must be isolated from the host with the disease and grown in pure culture.
- When a pure culture of the bacteria is inoculated into a healthy susceptible host, the specific disease must be reproduced.

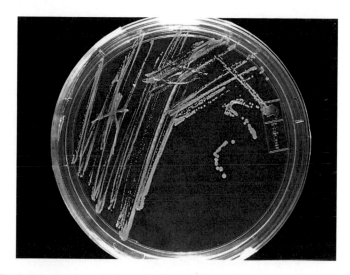

Fig. 7.6 Petri dish growing colonies of microorganisms. Source: U.S. National Oceanic and Atmospheric Administration. Public Domain. https://commons.wikimedia.org/wiki/File:Agar_plate_with_colonies.jpg

- The bacteria must be recoverable from the experimentally infected host and regrown in pure culture [6].

It may come as a surprise that Koch was not the first to propose this analytical process. These logical steps had previously been set forth in 1840 by German pathologist Friedrich Gustav Jakob Henle (1809–1885). But proof of the concept awaited Pasteur's discovery in the 1860s that germs cause disease, setting the stage for Koch and his stated postulates two decades later. Nevertheless, we honor Henle with the eponymous **Henle loop** in the kidney and the **Henle spine** in the mastoid area.

Not only postulates came from Koch and his associates. In this laboratory setting, a young microbiologist working as an assistant to Koch devised a mixture that included blood, carbohydrates, amino acids, and more, all in an agar base contained in a shallow plate. The laboratory assistant was Julius Richard Petri, and the **Petri dish** soon became indispensable in the microbiology laboratory (Fig. 7.6).

An Eponym Likely to Last

In ancient Greek, *lepros* meant scaly, and the word **leprosy** came to describe a number of skin diseases (Pepper, p. 128). It wasn't until the middle of the nineteenth century that use of the term came to be focused on the disease we associate with granulomatous deformities, public humiliation, and leper colonies.

Leprosy has been with us since prehistoric times, and Gould and Pyle (p. 911) theorize that a Roman army led by Pompey into Palestine carried the disease back to Europe. Over the centuries there was occasional confusion with syphilis, and some early cases that were described as leprosy may, in fact, have been syphilis. In those early days, both syphilis and leprosy were treated with the ever-popular remedy, mercury.

In 1873, Norwegian physician Gerhard Henrik Armauer Hansen (1841–1912) identified the causative agent, *Mycobacterium leprae*. This achievement made the organism the first bacterium identified as a specific cause of human disease. Today we honor Hansen with the eponymous **Hansen disease**, a name sure to survive the current anti-eponym furor, simply because it carries much less social stigma than the word leprosy (Fig. 7.7).

Tics and Sometimes Coprolalia

Tourette syndrome is an inherited disorder with multiple motor tics and at least one vocal tic, which sometimes involves **coprolalia**, from Greek *copros*, "excrement," and *lalia*, "talk, prattle." The word **coprolalia** was coined by the French neurologist Georges Gilles de la Tourette (1857–1904), who in 1825 described a case involving a noblewoman of his time [7].

Tourette was a student of French physician Jean-Martin Charcot (1825–1893), who named the disease **Gilles de la Tourette syndrome**. In 1893, Charcot died, and

Fig. 7.7 A 24-year-old man with Hansen disease/leprosy. Source: Pierre Arents. Public Domain. https://commons. wikimedia.org/wiki/ File:Leprosy.jpg

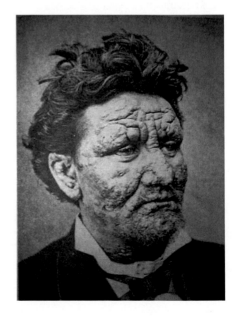

in that same year, Tourette was shot in the head by a former female patient who claimed—unlikely as it may sound—that he had hypnotized her against her will. Tourette began to experience mood swings and depression, and he died in a Swiss psychiatric hospital in 1904, at the age of 47.

Alzheimer Disease and Who Named It

In 1906, German physician Alois Alzheimer (1864–1915) described his patient, Auguste Deter, whom he had followed for five years as she experienced progressive memory loss and paranoia (Fig. 7.8). Following her death, he found severe atrophy of the brain with abnormal deposits in the nerve cells. Then in 1910, German psychiatrist and colleague of Alzheimer, Emil Kraepelin (1856–1926) published the eighth edition of his book *Psychiatrie*, in which we find the first use of the eponym **Alzheimer disease**.

Initially, the term **Alzheimer disease** described dementia in persons age 65 or less. Then in 1977, the meaning of the term was expanded to include persons of all ages.

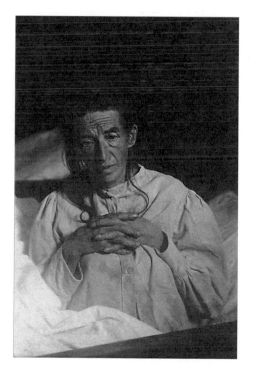

Fig. 7.8 Auguste Deter, the first described patient with Alzheimer Disease. Public Domain. https://commons.wikimedia.org/wiki/File:Auguste_D_aus_Marktbreit.jpg

The Tyranny of Alphabetization

In 1932, American gastroenterologist Burrill Bernard Crohn (1884–1983) and colleagues Leon Ginzburg and Gordon Oppenheimer published a report titled *Regional enteritis: a pathologic and clinical entity* [8]. History does not record who was principal investigator on this study, but we do find that the authors' names are listed alphabetically: *C*rohn, then *G*inzburg, finally *O*ppenheimer. Coincidence? I don't know, but today **regional enteritis** is often called **Crohn disease**. Might the disease have a different eponym if the unrecalled co-authors' names had started with letters earlier in the alphabet?

Sorry About that Nobel Prize

The **Papanicolaou test**, sometimes called the **Papanicolaou smear**, is a test introduced in the 1940s to screen for precancerous and cancerous disease of the uterine cervix. Its development is attributed to Greek physician Georgios Papanikolaou (1883–1962). Because of difficulty pronouncing the five-syllable surname, the process has become known as the **Pap test** or **Pap smear** (Fig. 7.9).

As with any preventive intervention, we will never know how many lives the Pap smear has saved, but it must be many. The clinical merits of the Pap smear led to Papanicolaou's nomination for a Nobel Prize in Physiology or Medicine. But there was an issue. It seems Romanian scientist Aurel Babeş (1886–1961), had devised a similar process in 1927. Upon finding that Papanicolaou had failed to cite the work of Babeş, the Nobel Prize bid was rejected [9].

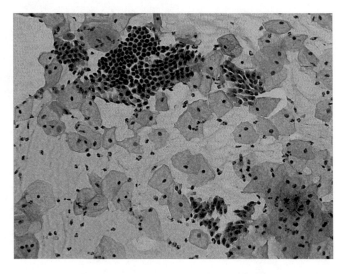

Fig. 7.9 Normal cervicovaginal cytology (pap smear). Source: Cagliostro~commonswiki. Public Domain. https://commons.wikimedia.org/wiki/File:Pap_test_wnl.jpg

The Peregrinating Problem Patient

Medical trainees learn about the **Munchausen syndrome**, and there was a real person behind the eponym: German cavalry officer Hieronymus Karl Friedrich Freiherr von Münchhausen (1720–1797). Upon his retirement von Münchhausen regaled all who would listen with tall tales of his adventures in the 1739 Russo-Turkish War.

Then in 1785, German writer Rudolph Erich Raspe (1736–1794) published a book titled *The Surprising Adventures of Baron Munchausen* (Fig. 7.10). Note the slightly different spelling of the name. The book was actually a work of political satire, but the stories caught on with the public, and the legend of the intrepid Baron was established (Gresham, p. 133). But the narrative was not yet medicalized.

Then, in 1951, British physician Richard Asher (1912–1965) published a description of a patient who wandered from one physician to another, describing worrisome symptoms suggesting devastating diseases. The author, recalling the tales of the Baron's exploits, coined the term **Munchausen syndrome** [10]. The disease is also sometimes dubbed the **hospital hopper syndrome**, the **hospital addiction syndrome**, the **tomomania syndrome**, and, in the days when patients actually had paper records, the **thick chart syndrome**.

Fig. 7.10 Baron
Munchausen. Public
Domain. https://commons.
wikimedia.org/wiki/
File:Fronta.gif

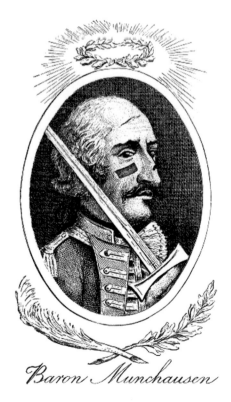

There is also a **Munchausen by proxy syndrome** in which caregivers fabricate illness or cause harm to someone in their care, often a child, all in an effort to gain attention or sympathy for themselves.

Eternal Life as a Cell Line

Can an acronym be an eponym? Perhaps it can, if more than just the first letters of the name are used. In 1951, a 31-year-old woman had carcinoma of the cervix, and a cell line harvested from that tumor site has yielded descendants employed extensively as a viral culture medium, including use in development of the Salk polio vaccine.

The cells are named **HeLa cells**, from the name of the source patient, Henrietta Lacks. The patient died in 1951, just months after the cells were obtained. The researcher who obtained the cells had neglected to obtain permission from Lacks for their use in science, and her descendants have received no royalties for their extensive use. The issues involved led to a 2010 book by Rebecca Skloot titled *The Immortal Life of Henrietta Lacks* (New York: Crown). A 2013 agreement with the National Institutes of Health allows family members a voice in how the HeLa cells will be used in research, but still no payments will be made.

With Approval of the Editor and the Down Family

The genetic disorder we know as **Down syndrome** has had several names. Because the root cause is the presence of all or part of a third copy of chromosome 21, it is known as **trisomy 21**. In 1846, French physician Édouard Séguin (1812–1880) coined the term **furfuraceous idiocy**, based on the Latin word for "scaly," presumably because of the dry, rough skin seen in many Down syndrome children. Today we remember the **Séguin signal**, an involuntary muscle contraction seen prior to an epileptic seizure.

The term **mongolism**, or **Mongoloid idiocy**, was introduced by British physician John Langdon Down (1828–1896). While serving as superintendent of the Royal Earlswood Asylum for Idiots in Surrey, Down found a series of patients with features which, he suggested, "might be a throwback to the Mongol racial type" (Porter, p. 587). The term mongolism persisted until its use by the World Health Organization (WHO) was challenged by the Mongolian delegation.

In 1961, several possible alternatives to mongolism were proposed to the editor of *The Lancet*. With approval of Down's family, the editor chose Down syndrome, with the comment:

> Down's Syndrome is an appropriate alternative for Mongoloid Idiocy until the chromosome abnormality in the disorder has been fully elucidated and a new scientific term has been coined.

The renaming of the genetic disorder was confirmed by the WHO in 1965 [11]. The current term used is, of course, the nonpossessive form.

About First Authors and Eponyms

In 1963, a report in *The Lancet* described a life-threatening syndrome of encephalopathy, liver involvement, and hyperammonemia [12] (Fig. 7.11). The syndrome has been associated with the use of aspirin by children during an otherwise mild viral illness. Currently the Centers for Disease Control and Prevention and other US government agencies recommend against the use of aspirin products in children under age 19 during bouts of febrile illness.

There were three authors on the paper, listed in reverse alphabetical order: Reye, Morgan, and Baral. Reye was first author, and hence the eponym **Reye syndrome**, honoring Australian pathologist Ralph Douglas Kenneth Reye (1912–1977). Who is listed first on key publications matters [13].

Eponymous Alice and Othello

Not all eponyms arose with actual, living persons. Some have come to us from literature and even the Bible.

In 1955, British psychiatrist John Todd (1914–1987) reported phenomena experienced by several of his migraine headache patients, who described seeing objects out of proportion and sometimes of sensing distorted perceptions of their own bod-

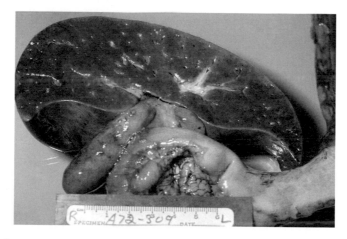

Fig. 7.11 Gross autopsy specimen of liver from child who died of Reye syndrome. Cut surface shows pallor due to fat accumulation in liver cells. Centers for Disease Control and Prevention. Public Domain. https://commons.wikimedia.org/wiki/File:66_lores.jpg

ies. In his report, Todd proposed that what his patients were describing mirrored events described by English writer Lewis Carroll (1832–1898) in his 1865 book *Alice's Adventures in Wonderland*. Todd's case was strengthened by the fact that in 1856, Carroll had consulted an ophthalmologist about the visual manifestations of his own migraine headaches [14].

The phenomenon has sometimes been called the **Todd syndrome**, after the man who first connected the disease manifestation and the young girl's adventures as described by Carroll, but it is better known as the **Alice in Wonderland syndrome**.

Todd, obviously widely read, also named the **Othello syndrome**, sometimes called **delusional jealousy** or **morbid jealousy** [15]. A person with the **Othello syndrome** becomes obsessed with the notion that his or her lover is unfaithful and acts out in harmful ways because of these ideas. The syndrome takes its name from Shakespeare's play *Othello*, in which the lead character kills his wife, Desdemona, whom he falsely believes has been adulterous (Fig. 7.12).

Being Forever Young

In 1890, Irish writer Oscar Wilde wrote a novel titled *The Picture of Dorian Gray*. The author tells of a man so self-absorbed with his image that upon viewing a portrait of himself, wishes that the picture, and not he, would suffer the ravages of aging. His wish is granted, but at the expense of his soul.

Then, in 2000, German psychotherapist Burkhard Brosig introduced the name of the novel's lead character to psychopathology in a paper presented at a symposium on the male quest for an eternally youthful body [16]. Today we sometimes see evidence of the **Dorian Gray syndrome** in aging movie stars and athletes who employ cosmetic procedures or performance-enhancing drugs in an effort to avoid aging.

I Won't Grow Up

Another literature-based eponym is the **Peter Pan syndrome**, popularized by American psychologist Dan Kiley in his book *The Peter Pan Syndrome: Men Who Have Never Grown Up* (New York: Dodd Mead, 1983). Based on the character created by Scottish playwright J. M. Barrie (1860–1937), a person with the Peter Pan syndrome has the body of an adult but the emotional maturity of a child (Fig. 7.13). He, and it is usually a male, or she just does not seem to grow up. The *Urban Dictionary* uses the word "manolescent" to describe this type of man. Somehow the name Michael Jackson comes to mind.

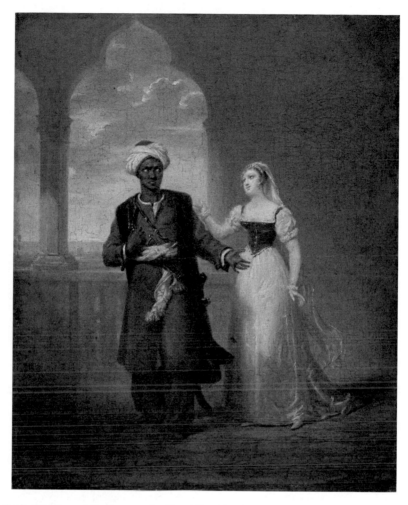

Fig. 7.12 Othello and Desdemona, by Henri Jean-Baptiste Victoire Fradelle, ca. 1827. Source: Folger Shakespeare Library Digital Image Collection. Public Domain. https://commons.wikimedia.org/wiki/File:Othello_and_Desdemona_(Fradelle,_c.1827).jpg

In his book, Kiley also gave us the term **Wendy Syndrome**, describing the enabling mother figure who empowers the irresponsibility of the Peter Pan figure. In today's lingo we have the **helicopter parent,** hovering above an over-protected child.

The **Cinderella syndrome,** named for the fairy-tale heroine, describes a woman who is productive, supportive, and loveable, but is abused by her female peers and who can only be rescued from her dilemma by an outside agent—Prince Charming. The syndrome, sometimes called the **Cinderella complex,** is described in the 1981 book *The Cinderella Complex: Women's Hidden Fear of Independence* (New York: Simon & Schuster) by American psychotherapist Colette Dowling (born 1938).

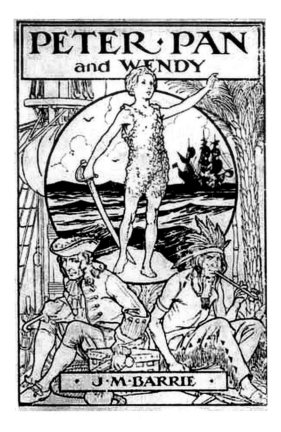

Popeye, Orphan Annie, and Satchmo

Popular culture affords us many descriptive terms. In the medical literature, we find reports of the **Popeye syndrome**, hypertrophy of the muscles of the upper extremity owing to heavy work (Fig. 7.14). Enlargement of the forearms, resembling those of the comic strip character Popeye, so that they are relatively larger that the upper arms, can cause entrapment of the brachial artery [17].

The **Little Orphan Annie-eye** nuclear inclusion is a classic histopathological observation describing large nuclei with cleared centers, found in patients with papillary cancer of the thyroid. The allusion is credited to Dr. Nancy E. Warner of the University of Southern California and harkens to the vacuous eyes of the orphan girl in the daily comic strip *Little Orphan Annie* by American cartoonist Harold Gray (1894–1968).

In 1935, Louis "Satchmo" Armstrong was forced to stop playing the trumpet for a year because of increasing weakness in the muscles of his lips, which resulted in an inability to maintain high notes. Today we have the **Satchmo syndrome**, a rupture of the orbicularis oris muscle, found in musicians who play trumpet and other brass instruments requiring high pressure to achieve their best music.

Fig. 7.14 Popeye, East
Hampton, New York.
Credit: Tomás Fano.
Creative Commons. https://
commons.wikimedia.org/
wiki/File:New_York._
East_Hampton._Popeye_
(2710256517).jpg

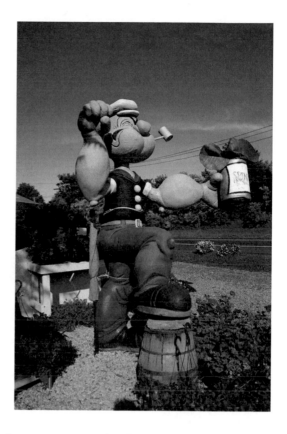

These three culturally derived eponyms may also be considered *augenblick* **diagnoses**. In German *augenblick* means "blink of the eye." Examples include the bulging eyes of Graves disease, the shuffling gait and limited mobility of parkinsonism, and the persistent hoarseness of laryngeal paralysis, although the latter might better be described by another German word, *hörenkurz*, meaning to "hear shortly."

In a generation will anyone recall Popeye, Orphan Annie, or Satchmo? Will these terms cause future young physicians to roll their eyes and scratch their heads?

A Biblical Eponym

In 1966, Davis et al. described two girls with recurrent staphylococcal abscesses accompanied by chronic dermatitis and pneumonias [18]. Recalling the Biblical prophet Job, whose body Satan covered with boils, the authors named the disease **Job's syndrome**. Also called **hyper IgE syndrome** because of high serum levels of IgE, it is a rare disorder, affecting both sexes, that typically begins in childhood.

Autoeponyms, Baseball, and the Iron Horse

A medical disorder named for an individual who was affected by, and often died of, the disease is called an **autoeponym**. Although the emerging style is to omit the possessive when a condition is named for a physician or scientist who described it, diseases named for patients are often, but not always, expressed using the possessive form.

One of the best-known autoeponymous diseases is **Lou Gehrig's disease**, named for American baseball player Lou Gehrig, actually born Heinrich Ludwig Gehrig (1903–1941) (Fig. 7.15). During his major league baseball career, lasting from 1923 through 1939, Gehrig received the nickname "The Iron Horse" for playing in 2130 consecutive games, a record finally surpassed in 1995 by Cal Ripken, Jr. Gehrig's career was cut short when he developed **amyotrophic lateral sclerosis**, which progressed to claim his life in 1941 [19].

The Truth About Pott's Fracture

Although not often used today, the term **Pott's fracture** describes a bimalleolar fracture of the ankle. The injury was described by English surgeon Percivall Pott (1714–1788) in his 1769 monograph *Some Few Remarks upon Fractures and Dislocations*, 4 years after he sustained a serious fracture of the lower extremity in a fall from his horse in London.

Fig. 7.15 Lou Gehrig during his major league baseball rookie year, 1923. Author: Wide World Photos. Public Domain. https://commons. wikimedia.org/wiki/ File:1923_Lou_Gehrig.png

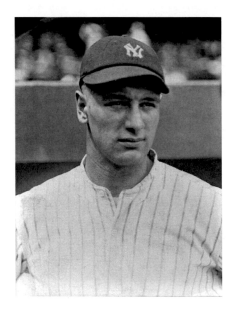

Following his fracture, and fearful that being moved by carriage from the injury site to a hospital might aggravate the injury and lead to amputation, Pott had two men create a makeshift litter from two poles and a door and take him to his home. Amputation was considered, but in the end, the injury was splinted and the patient recovered. As a historical curiosity, Pott's injury was actually an open tibial fracture and not the bimalleolar ankle fracture that today bears his name.

The Hunterian Chancre of Syphilis

The true, hard chancre that represents the initial stage of syphilis is called the **Hunterian chancre**, an autoeponym traced to Scottish surgeon John Hunter (1728–1793) (Fig. 7.16). Although some question the story, Sebastian (p. 405) describes how, in studying venereal disease about the year 1750, Hunter inoculated himself with the pus from a patient with gonorrhea. Unfortunately the donor also had syphilis, and the surgeon went on to develop manifestations of syphilis, including—perhaps—luetic aortitis and neurosyphilis.

More Diseases Named for Patients

In his first-ever medical scientific paper, published in 1798, English physicist John Dalton (1766–1844) described his own red-green colorblindness, the first formal report of the visual abnormality [20]. Dirckx (p. 82) tells that Dalton's extreme colorblindness led to his sometimes wearing clothes "whose hues scandalized his fellow Quakers." Today, **daltonism** is occasionally used as a synonym for red-green colorblindness.

Another autoeponymous entity is **Thomsen's disease**, describing episodic muscle spasms, with impaired ability to relax muscles normally, also called **myotonia congenita**. This type of myotonia was first described by Danish/German physician Asmus Julius Thomsen (1815–1896), who told of his own manifestations of the disease and those of his family members in 1876.

English physician Jonathan Hutchinson (1828–1913) is credited with first describing, in 1898, a spreading dermatitis that came to be called **Mortimer's disease** to honor Hutchinson's patient, Mrs. Mortimer. At times the term **Mortimer's disease** or **Mortimer's malady** has also been used as a synonym for sarcoidosis.

Hemophilia B, a genetically transmitted clotting disorder involving a deficiency of factor IX, is also called **Christmas disease**, named for Stephen Christmas. Stephen was the youngest of seven patients with the rare disease first reported in the December 1952 issue of the *British Medical Journal* (BMJ). Was the report being published in the Christmas issue of the BMJ a coincidence or another example of subtle British humor?

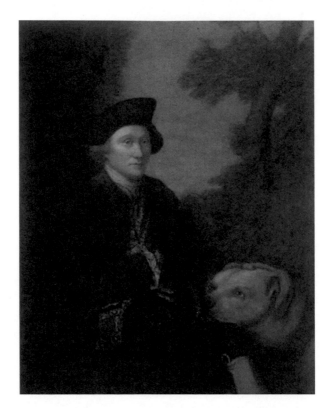

Fig. 7.16 Portrait of John Hunter. By Dorofield Hardy, a copy of the original by Robert Home now in the Royal Society, ca. 1770. Public Domain. https://commons.wikimedia.org/wiki/File:Hardy_-_John_Hunter_(after_Home).png

Hartnup disease, a hereditary disorder causing a pellagra-like dermatitis, cerebellar ataxia, and gross aminoaciduria, named for the Hartnup family of London, was described in a 1956 paper by Baron et al. [21].

Where Some Drug Names Originated

When a child named Margaret Tracy suffered an open fracture of the leg in 1943, before the widespread availability of penicillin and the other antibiotics that would eventually follow, an infection developed. An organism cultured from the child's wound—*Bacillus subtilis*—produced a polypeptide with antimicrobial properties. The antibiotic produced, and still used today, was named **bacitracin**: *baci–* for "bacillus," and *–tracin*, after the girl with the infected wound.

Warfarin (Coumadin) began as a rodenticide. Following studies to determine the cause of bleeding in cattle ingesting spoiled hay made from sweet clover, scientists at the University of Wisconsin discovered the anticoagulant warfarin, marketed

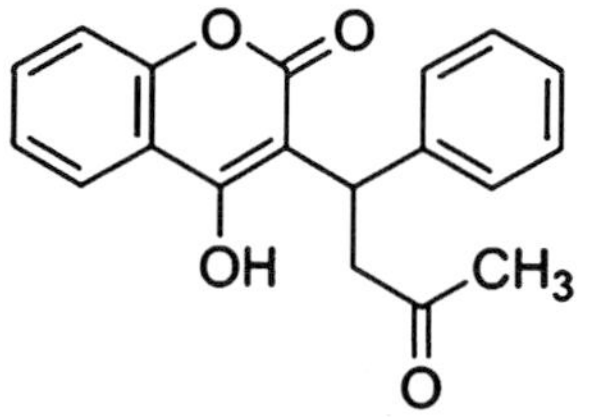

Fig. 7.17 Chemical
structure of warfarin.
Author: Emeldir. Public
Domain. https://commons.
wikimedia.org/wiki/
File:4-hydroxy-3-(3-oxo-1-
phenylbutyl)-2H-chromen-
2-one_200.svg

in 1948 to kill mice and rats (Fig. 7.17). The drug took its name from the laboratory's funding source: Wisconsin Alumni Research Foundation—WARF—combined with *–arin*, from the known anticoagulant, **coumarin**. The hint that the drug might be clinically useful occurred in 1951, as a young soldier attempted suicide using warfarin. He was treated with the specific antidote, vitamin K, but the incident suggested that the drug might be clinically effective when anticoagulation was needed.

Nystatin (Mycostatin) is an antifungal agent that can be used topically, orally, or vaginally. The drug, like many antimicrobials, came from a species of bacteria. The source was the soil of a farm owned by a family named Nourse. The organism was dubbed *Streptomyces noursei* by American scientists Elizabeth Lee Hazen (1885–1975) and Rachel Fuller Brown (1898–1980), working in the New York State Health Department Laboratory. When Hazen and Brown developed the antifungal drug in 1954, they named it **nystatin** to honor their laboratory: *ny–* for New York, *–stat* for state, plus *–in*.

A drug name may honor an animal, as well as a human. **Ursodeoxycholic acid**, or **ursodiol**, is a bile acid used to treat various liver diseases. The name comes from the Latin *ursa*, "bear," because the active substance in the drug is found in bear bile.

Smoldering Eponymous Controversies

Some calls to eliminate well-known eponyms arise from historical facts that have come to light involving the physicians and scientists whose names have been dishonored. Here are three of those.

Reiter syndrome, named for German physician Hans Conrad Julius Reiter (1881–1969), is an autoimmune response to an infection, leading to the classic triad of conjunctivitis, urethritis, and arthritis, giving us the mnemonic: can't see, can't pee, and can't climb a tree. According to Matteson et al., Reiter was an early convert to Nazism and served as president of the German Health Ministry, with direct oversight of the Nazi racial hygiene program that resulted in the deaths of countless "undesirables" (Fig. 7.18). There is a current tendency to use the term **reactive arthritis**, although this phrase does not include two of the three classic manifestations of the disease [22].

Fig. 7.18 Hans Conrad
Julius Reiter. Author:
Ahmed H. Elbestawey.
Creative Commons. https://
commons.wikimedia.org/
wiki/File:Hans-Reiter.jpg

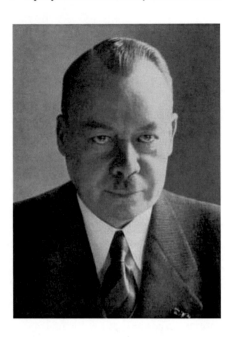

Another eponym under the cloud of activities during World War II is **Wegener granulomatosis**, named for German pathologist Friedrich Wegener (1907–1990). It turns out that Wegener was a Nazi who also supported the Nazi racial hygiene program [22]. There is speculation that his activities involved experiments on death camp inmates. The American College of Chest Physicians (ACCP) awarded Wegener a "master clinician" prize in 1989, which was withdrawn when his wartime activities came to light in 2000. Today the preferred name of the disease is **granulomatosis with polyangiitis.**

Austrian physician Hans Asperger (1906–1980) was instrumental in developing the theory of autism. However, in their book *In a Different Key: The Story of Autism*, Donovan and Zucker suggest that Asperger may have been a Nazi collaborator whose subjects were later sent to be euthanized. If confirmed, this allegation would place the eponymous **Asperger syndrome** in jeopardy [23].

Introduction to Tashima's Syndrome

In 1965, American oncologist Charles K. Tashima identified a new syndrome described as "a condition in which a physician searches for a new sign, disease, or syndrome to which his name can be attached" [24]. Since the author apparently suffered the syndrome himself, this seems to be an autoeponym: **Tashima's syndrome.** This means that all who first identified backpacker's diarrhea, skier's thumb, and runner's knee missed their chances for eponymous immortality.

References

1. Board Question 70965. Available at: https://theboard.byu.edu/questions/70935/
2. Woywodt A, et al. Should eponyms be abandoned? Yes. BMJ. 2007;335:424.
3. Chadwick J, Mann WN (trans.) Hippocratic writings. Harmondsworth, UK: Penguin; 1978:170.
4. Hughes JT. Eponymists in medicine. London: Royal Society of Medicine Services; 1991.
5. Addison T. On the constitutional and local effects of disease of the suprarenal capsules. London: Samuel Highley;1855.
6. Definition of Koch's postulates. MedicineNet.com. Available at: http://www.medicinenet.com/script/main/art.asp?articlekey=7105
7. Itard JMG. *Mémoire sur quelques functions involontaires des appareils de la locomotion, de la préhension et de la voix.* Arch Gen Med. 1825;8:385.
8. Crohn BB, et al. Regional enteritis: a pathologic and clinical entity. Mount Sinai J Med. 1932;67:263.
9. Koss LG, Aurel Babes. Int J Gynecol Path. 2003;22:101.
10. Asher R. Munchausen's syndrome. Lancet. 1951; 1(6650):339.
11. Ward OC. John Langdon Down: the man and the message. Down Syndr Res Pract. 1999;6:19.
12. Reye RD, et al. Encephalopathy and fatty degeneration of the viscera. Lancet. 1963;2:749.
13. Taylor RB. What every medical writer needs to know. New York: Springer: 2015.
14. Todd J. The syndrome of Alice in Wonderland. Can Med Assn J. 1955;73:701.
15. Todd J, et al. The Othello syndrome: a study in the psychopathology of sexual jealousy. J Nervous Ment Dis. 1955;122:367.
16. Brosig B. The "Dorian Gray syndrome" and other fountains of youth. Paper presented at the Continuous Medical Education Board of the Landesärztekammer Hessen, Clinical Pharmacology Section, on 29.4.2000 in Bad Nauheim, FRG.
17. Biemans RG. The Popeye syndrome—brachial artery entrapment as a result of muscular hypertrophy. Neth J Surg. 1984;36:103.
18. Davis S, et al. Job's syndrome: recurrent, "cold", staphylococcal abscesses. Lancet. 1966;1:1013.
19. Graham F. Lou Gehrig: A quiet hero. Boston: Houghton Mifflin, 1969.
20. Dalton J. Extraordinary facts relating to the vision of colours, with observation. Mem Literary Philos Soc Manchester. 1798;5:28.
21. Baron DN, et al. Hereditary pellagra-like skin rash with temporary cerebellar ataxia, constant renal aminoaciduria, and other bizarre biochemical features. Lancet. 1956;271:421.
22. Matteson EL. Eponymophilia in rheumatology. Rheumatology. 2006;45:1328.
23. Donovan J, Zucker C. In a different key: the story of autism. New York: Crown; 2016.
24. Tashima CK. Tashima's syndrome. JAMA. 1965;194:208

Chapter 8
Medical Authorisms and Their Creators

An **authorism** is a word made up by a writer, an attributable neologism, and there are many in the medical dictionary. I hold that an authorism isn't legitimate unless two criteria are met: the first is that the word "catches on" and that it is adapted and continues in use. This is in contrast to a **nonce word**, one created to solve a need to communicate for a single occasion, but that never becomes accepted and used later. The term nonce word was coined by Sir James Augustus Henry Murray (1837–1915), editor of the *Oxford English Dictionary*. In Murray's dictionary we find the nonce words **twi-thought**, **witchcraftical**, and **touch-me-not-ishness**, all of which make perfect sense to me even if I don't see them in books today. The single-purpose word **supercalifragilisticexpialidocious**, from the movie *Mary Poppins*, is familiar to most of us. Sometimes one-time words are reborn: the word **quark** began as a nonce word in James Joyce's *Finnegans Wake* in the phrase "Three quarks for Muster Mark!" In 1964, it was adapted by American physicist Murray Gell-Mann (born 1929) as the name of very tiny building blocks of matter that combine to form protons and neutrons.

The second criterion for authorism is that we can identify the creator with reasonable certainty. English physician Sir Thomas Browne (1605–1682), author of *Religio Medici* (The Religion of the Physician), gave us **locomotion**, **ambidextrous**, and **suicide**. We can attribute **streptococcus** to Austrian surgeon Albert Theodor Billroth (1829–1894), and Scottish surgeon and scientist Alexander Ogston (1844–1929) gave us **staphylococcus**. It was Swiss psychiatrist Carl Jung (1875–1961), and not Sigmund Freud, who named a psychological problem a **complex** (Forsyth, p. 53). The word **microalbuminuria** entered our clinical vocabulary in 1964, created by English physician Harry Keen (1925–2013).

Not all authorisms are created by physicians and scientists. America's third president, Thomas Jefferson (1743–1826), gave us the verb **to neologize**, as well as the words **pedicure**, **indecipherable**, and **electioneering**. According to Forsyth (p. 111), when English romantic poet Percy Bysshe Shelley "couldn't think of a word he just made one up." Shelley's neologisms include **heartless**, **expressionless**, **optimistic**, **expatriate**, and **national anthem**.

R.B. Taylor, *The Amazing Language of Medicine*,
DOI 10.1007/978-3-319-50328-8_8

149

Most authorisms that have filled a need—such as **anesthesia** and **pellagra**—have become legitimate entries in the medical dictionary. A few, covered at the end of the chapter, represent the clinical slang often used by medical trainees.

Not all authorisms survive. Here are three that are lost is the mists of lexicographical history:

* Sir Thomas Browne, mentioned above, gave us the word **balneation**, meaning bathing.
* In 1851, American physician Samuel A. Cartwright (1793–1863) coined the term **drapetomania**, describing a mental aberration compelling black slaves to flee to freedom.
* British physician and author Havelock Ellis (1859–1839) proposed the term **homogenic** as preferable to the word homosexual. The word he proposed is used today in genetics, where it has another meaning entirely. The current alternative to homosexual seems to be *gay*.

Tones and Tonics in Music and Health

Pythagoras (570–489 BCE) was a Greek philosopher, and his teaching gave us the Pythagoreans, whose interests included both medicine and music. According to Koestler, "they used medicine to purge the body, and music to purge the soul" [1]. They used the word *tonikos*, meaning stretching, in the sense that the body had cords composed of earth, air, fire, and water that needed to be maintained in proper tone. Thus—more or less—from Pythagoras, we get our word **tonic**.

From here the path takes some odd turns. Over the years, the word tonic often described a few herbs dissolved in an alcohol base. A popular one was Peruna, a tonic manufactured in Ohio by Dr. Samuel Hartman in the early 1900s, based on the assertion that "catarrhal grip" was widespread in America and that Peruna—with 28 percent alcohol content—can cure the affliction. Then there was Hadacol, a collection of vitamins in 12 percent alcohol, the latter identified as a "preservative."

So-called **tonic water**, or **Indian tonic water**, describes quinine in water consumed by the British in India to prevent malaria, beginning in the nineteenth century. Because quinine in water is quite bitter, the resourceful Brits began to add distilled spirits to the mixture, giving us our now-popular beverage, gin and tonic (Fig. 8.1).

In the late 1950s, a favorite compound was Ritonic, containing methyltestosterone, ethinyl estradiol, assorted vitamins and minerals, and—notably—the stimulant methylphenidate (Ritalin), recommended "for patients who are losing their drive, alertness, vitality and zest for living because of the natural degenerative changes of advancing years" [2]. Ritonic was taken off the market in 1962, a great disappointment to many patients.

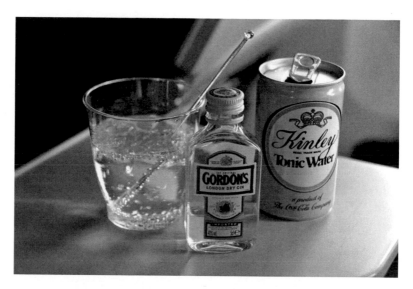

Fig. 8.1 Gin and tonic. Source: cyclonebill from Copenhagen, Denmark. Creative Commons. https://commons.wikimedia.org/wiki/File:Gin_%26_tonic_(4621166646).jpg

That Which Stands Before

A century and a half after Pythagoras, the Greek physician Erasistratus (304–250 BCE), together with his physician colleague Herophilus, taught medicine and studied anatomy in Alexandria. Although he had a special interest in the brain, we mention Erasistratus here as the father of the word **prostate**. He both described the organ and gave it its current name.

In ancient Greek the word *prostates* means a guard, one who "stands before." Yes, the prostate does stand before the bladder, but many older men wish the gland would be a little less vigilant and be more lenient in allowing the flow of urine from the bladder. According to Kovner, Erasistratus invented the urinary catheter, presumably as part of his study of the **prostate gland** [3] .

The Rectum: First or Last

Upon finding the last part of the intestine of animals to be straight, a Greek physician in the Roman Empire, Claudius Galen (129–200), named it the **rectum**, from the Latin word meaning "straight." Of course, when it comes to humans, the distal portion of the large intestine is a continuation of the sigmoid colon that begins at the level of the third sacral vertebrae and ends at the anal canal; it really isn't straight at all.

Before Galen, Hippocrates (ca. 460–377 BCE) called the terminal colon the *archos*, from a Greek word meaning "chief" or "first." Think of archbishop, the "first" among the bishops, or perhaps of archangel, archenemy, or archetype. The "arch" applied to the lowest part of the large intestine later became *arsch* in German, and eventually *arse*, once a respectable term in the English language (Pepper, p. 32).

Insane, Insanity, and Bedlam

Our word **insane** is the current iteration of the Latin *insanus*, from *in–* and *sanus*, meaning "not" and "healthy." The medical use of the term **insanity**, *insania*, was in the third book of *De Medicina*, by Roman encyclopedist Aurelius Cornelius Celsus (ca. 25 BCE–ca 50 CE), written during the reign of Tiberius Caesar. In 1478, the eight-volume book became one of the first medical books to be printed (Garrison, p. 107).

Over the centuries we have seen variable approaches to the diagnosis and treatment of the insane. Hippocrates saw insanity as an illness caused by an excess of black bile. In the later Roman era, those with mental illness were treated humanely and even afforded leniency for criminal acts. Treatment became harsher during medieval times, and in the Bethlehem Royal Hospital in London, founded in 1247 and the source of our current word **bedlam**, patients were often restrained with ropes and chains (Fig. 8.2). The word Bethlehem comes from Hebrew *Beth-lehem*, "House of Bread" (Train, p. 13).

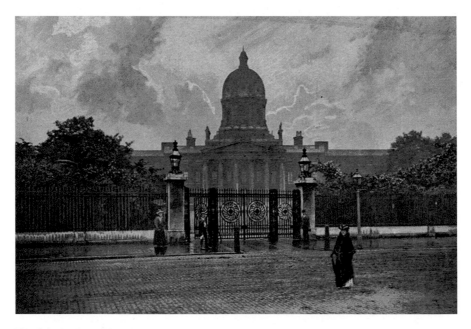

Fig. 8.2 A view of Bethlehem Royal Hospital, London, from Lambeth Road, published before 1896. Public Domain. https://commons.wikimedia.org/wiki/File:Bethlam_1896.gif

Today insanity is a legal term in the United States; health professionals use more specific diagnoses such as schizophrenia and organic brain syndrome.

In Praise of Laudanum

Laudanum is an alcohol-based solution of opium alkaloids, better known today as tincture of opium. Swiss-German alchemist Philippus Aureolus Theophrastus Bombastus von Hohenheim, better known as Paracelsus (1493–1541), is credited with first combining opium and alcohol, and for giving it the name laudanum, probably from the Latin *laudare*, "to praise" (Onions, p. 517) (Fig. 8.3).

In the seventeenth century, English physician Thomas Sydenham (1624–1689) concocted his own laudanum formula, which contained not only opium but also saffron, cinnamon, cloves, and sherry wine. There have been other formulas, with varying percentages of alcohol.

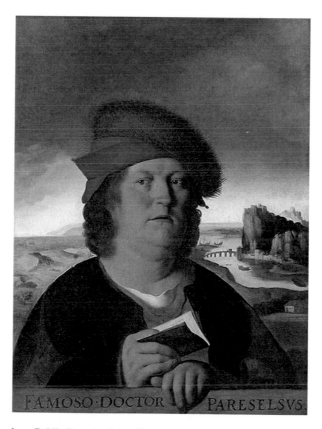

Fig. 8.3 Paracelsus. Public Domain. https://commons.wikimedia.org/wiki/File:Paracelsus.jpg

In the past, classic laudanum—**tincture of opium**—was used for many reasons, including pain, insomnia, cough, heart disease, and even meningitis. Prior to the Harrison Narcotics Tax Act of 1914, the compound, cheaper than a bottle of gin, was a widely used recreational substance. It is still occasionally used to treat intractable diarrhea, and early in my rural practice years, I prescribed tincture of opium when nothing else seemed to control protracted diarrhea.

The Sheath and the Sword

The word **vagina** in Latin means "sheath" or "scabbard." Italian physician Gabriele Falloppio (1523–1562) was first to use the word to name the canal in females that connects the uterine cervix with the outside world (Garrison, p. 223).

On the other hand, **penis** in Latin means "tail," clearly an etymologic misperception, although Rawson (p. 296) tells, "To the Romans, the *penis* was a *gladius*, or 'sword.'" The Roman image fits much better with the vagina being a "sheath" or "scabbard." Rawson also points out that the word vagina entered the Oxford English Dictionary in 1682, two years before acceptance of the word penis.

Jail, Camp, and Ship Fever

In the days of Hippocrates, *typhos* meant "smoke" or "stupor," a reasonable description of the mental status of many with acute febrile disease. The disease **typhus** is just such an illness, caused by rickettsial bacteria and spread by lice, fleas, or ticks. It had a historically significant impact on Napoleon's ill-advised 1812 invasion into Russia. Typhus has sometimes been described by the setting in which it occurs: **jail fever**, **camp fever**, **ship fever**, **hospital fever**, or **famine fever**. Other colorful terms for typhus were **putrid fever** and **pestilential fever**.

The disease typhus was so named in 1760 by French physician and botanist François Boissier de Sauvages (1710–1767), honored today with the botanical term *Sauvagesia*, the name of a genus of plants in family *Ochnaceae*.

Angina Pectoris and Cordis

English physician William Heberden (1710–1801) created the term **angina pectoris** in 1768 (Fig. 8.4). In his paper he wrote of a "disorder of the breast." **Angina** comes from the Latin *angere*, to "strangle." Roman playwright Plautus (ca. 254–184 BC) used the word to describe an abscess of the tonsils, what we now sometimes call quinsy (Maleska, p. 66). And there is **Ludwig angina**, a rapidly progressive cellulitis of the floor of the mouth, named for the German physician who published the first description of the condition in 1836, Wilhelm von Ludwig (1790–1865).

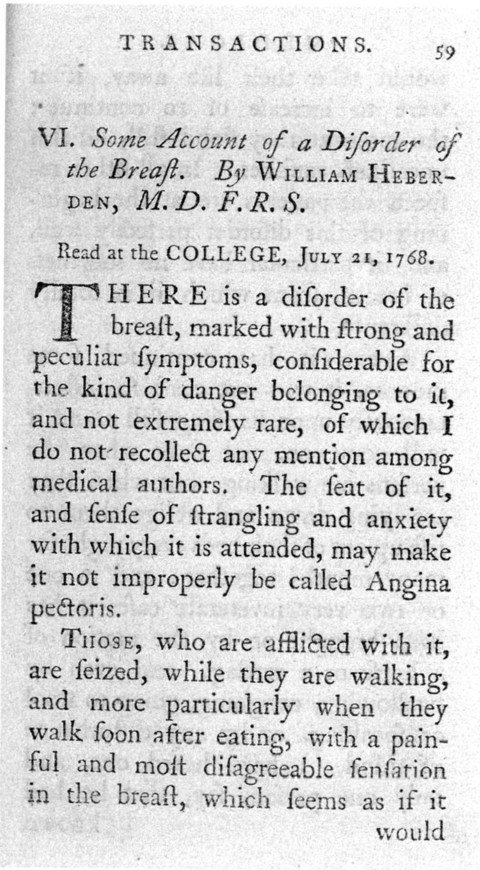

Fig. 8.4 William
Heberden, Account of a
disorder of the breast.
Source: Wellcome Images.
Public Domain. https://
commons.wikimedia.org/
wiki/File:Heberden,_
Account_of_a_disorder_
of_the_breast,_1772_
Wellcome_L0009915.jpg

TRANSACTIONS.   59

VI. *Some Account of a Diſorder of
the Breaſt.* By WILLIAM HEBER-
DEN, *M. D. F. R. S.*

Read at the COLLEGE, JULY 21, 1768.

THERE is a diſorder of the
breaſt, marked with ſtrong and
peculiar ſymptoms, conſiderable for
the kind of danger belonging to it,
and not extremely rare, of which I
do not recollect any mention among
medical authors. The ſeat of it,
and ſenſe of ſtrangling and anxiety
with which it is attended, may make
it not improperly be called Angina
pectoris.

THOSE, who are afflicted with it,
are ſeized, while they are walking,
and more particularly when they
walk ſoon after eating, with a painful and moſt diſagreeable ſenſation
in the breaſt, which ſeems as if it
would

When it came time to name his new syndrome, I find it interesting that Heberden
wrote of the "breast," and used "pectoris," from the Latin form *pectus*, pertaining to
the chest, as if he may not have connected the pain to the heart at all. A more precise
term would have been *angina cordis,* from the Latin *cor*, meaning heart.

Diarrhea, Dementia, and Dermatitis

Pellagra is a deficiency of niacin, also called vitamin B3, and is classically found in
persons whose food consists chiefly of corn products, or whose diets are otherwise
deficient in sources of niacin such as fish, meat, and vegetables. Following the introduction of corn, or maize, into Europe, pellagra became common among those who
could not afford a more diverse diet.

The disease has three classic features—diarrhea, dementia, and dermatitis. Death
can be the fourth manifestation. In 1753, Catalan physician Gaspar Casal (1681–
1759) described the disease, calling it *mal de rosa* (Garrison, p. 368), a Spanish

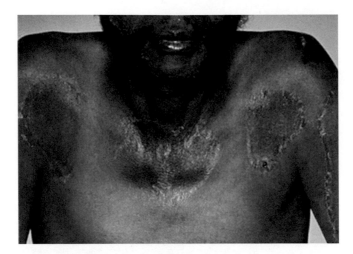

Fig. 8.5 Skin lesions of pellagra. Credit: Herbert L. Fred, MD; Hendrik A. van Dijk. Creative Commons. https://commons.wikimedia.org/wiki/File:Pellagra3.jpg

phrase that means "bad pink." Casal's name has been linked to the disease in regard to the dermatitis; a patient with pellagra may have a **Casal collar** or **Casal necklace**, referring to an erythematous rash in the C3–C4 dermatomes.

Then in 1771, Italian physician Francesco Frapolli described a condition then common in northern Italy, giving it the name **pellagra**, from the Italian *pelle agra*, meaning "rough skin" (Ackerknecht, p. 148) (Fig. 8.5).

Pellagra was a problem in the United States, especially in the Southeast, and was one of the causes of the high death rates in southern prison camps during the 1861–1865 Civil War (Bordley and Harvey, p. 248). The disease remained a problem until 1916, when American public health physician, Joseph Goldberger (1874–1929), identified its cause, prompting recommendations to encourage the inclusion of vitamin-containing vegetables and fruits in the diet.

From Stone to Soft Drink

The Greek word *lithos*, meaning "stone," is the source of our term **lithium**, a metallic element named in 1818 by Swedish chemist Jöns Jacob Berzelius (1779–1848). The name was chosen to clarify that the source of the element was mineral, in contradistinction to other elements of vegetable or animal origin.

Over the years lithium has had many uses, including in the production of soaps, lubricating greases, batteries, and nuclear weapons. In the past, it was prescribed to treat arthritis, gout, and uremia—all with more harm than benefit. Then the serendipitous discovery that the injection of a **lithium salt** into guinea pigs caused sedation led to its eventual use in the treatment of bipolar disorder (Li, p. 140).

Lithium has also been an ingredient in a soft drink. What we now know as *7UP* began in 1929 as *Bib-Label Lithiated Lemon-Lime Soda*, with the catchy slogan: "Takes the 'ouch' out of grouch." Lithium was listed as an ingredient on the bottle label from the product's beginning until it was removed from the drink in 1948. Although we are not sure, the name 7UP may have indicated the drink's original seven ingredients, or referred to the presence of lithium, which has an atomic mass of about seven. Whatever the source of the name, the lithium in the beverage may have actually have had medicinal value for some persons with bipolar disorder.

Like Curing and Preventing Like

Homeopathy is a system of alternative medicine based on the principle that substances that cause disease manifestations can cure such manifestations when they are part of an illness. The approach to medical care and the word homeopathy were the brainchild of German physician Samuel Hahnemann (1755–1843) who held that "like cures like," or, perhaps more impressively in Latin, *similia similibus curantur* (Fig. 8.6). The word comes from Greek *homoios*, "similar, like," and *patheis*, "disease." In his system of medicine, Hahnemann recommended very tiny amounts of substances, often plant based, to treat disease.

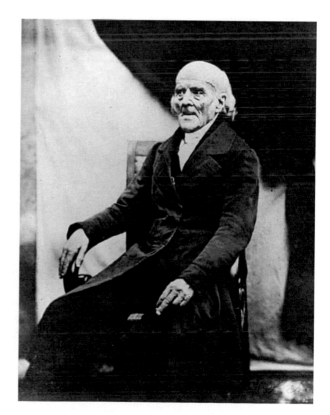

Fig. 8.6 Daguerreotype of Samuel Hahnemann, 1841. Public Domain. https://commons.wikimedia.org/wiki/File:Samuel_Hahnemann_1841.jpg

Although it would be a stretch to say that homeopathy is mainstream medicine today, the idea that minute quantities of a disease-causing substance—poliovirus, for example—might *prevent* later disease is the basis of much that we do in preventive medicine. Like doesn't cure like, but can prevent it. We call this **immunization**.

The Path to Painless Surgery

Paracelsus studied the hypnotic effects of ether in the sixteenth century. British chemist Michael Faraday (1791–1867) was well familiar with the consciousness-altering properties of the gas, owing to his participation in "ether parties" [4]. Then in 1841, American rural physician Crawford Long used ether to allow the painless removal of a patient's neck tumor, charging two dollars for the surgery and 25 cents for the ether. But, alas, Long neither published his success nor did he coin a neologism.

In 1846, **American dentist William T. G. Morton (1819–1868)** demonstrated the effectiveness of ether anesthesia in the surgical amphitheater of Massachusetts General Hospital, now called the "Ether Dome" (Li, p. 194) (Fig. **8.7**). As was the case with Long, the patient's problem was a tumor of the neck. The surgery and the

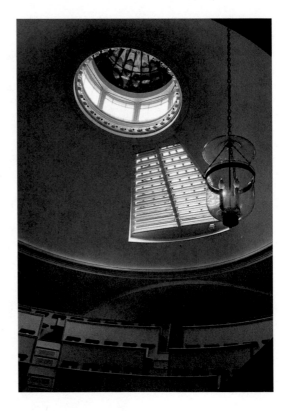

Fig. 8.7 The Ether Dome at the top of the Bulfinch Building at Massachusetts General Hospital in Boston, MA as photographed on 27 July 2013. Credit: Ravi Poorun [oddityinabox]. Creative Commons. https://commons.wikimedia.org/wiki/File:Inside_the_Ether_Dome_-_27_July_2013.jpg

pain control were both successful, the triumph was reported in print, and Morton is today credited with introducing anesthesia to the world of medicine. But it was American physician and scholar Oliver Wendell Holmes (1809–1894) who in 1846 gave us the word **anesthesia**, derived from the Greek *anaisthesia*, "lack of sensation."

Fear of the Marketplace

Anxiety when faced with crowds is called **agoraphobia**, from the Greek words *agora*, meaning "open space," connoting the marketplace, and *phobia*, "fear." The patient has an excessive fear of being in public and may become housebound. The word was created in 1871 by German psychiatrist Carl Friedrich Otto Westphal (1833–1890). He is eponymously remembered today for the **Westphal sign**, the absence of the patellar tendon reflex seen in various diseases of the spinal cord or brain.

Some famous persons believed to have suffered agoraphobia include French author, mathematician, and philosopher Blaise Pascal (1623–1662); English naturalist Charles Darwin (1809–1882); and American poet Emily Dickinson (1830–1886).

Appendicitis and its Named Signs

The word **appendicitis** comes from Latin *appendix*, meaning "something attached," and –*itis*, "inflammation." American physician Reginald Heber Fitz (1843–1913) coined the word in 1886, when he recognized that the abscesses frequently seen in the right iliac fossa were caused by perforating inflammation of the vermiform ("worm-shaped") appendix. Although Fitz is not the source of any eponym I can find, the appendix and the inflammation thereof have given us many named clinical signs. Here are a few:

- **McBurney sign** is tenderness at McBurney point on the right side of the abdomen, named for American surgeon Charles McBurney (1845–1913).
- A **Rovsing sign**, after Danish surgeon Niels Thorkild Rovsing (1862–1927), is positive when palpation deeply in the left lower quadrant evokes pain in the right lower quadrant of the abdomen.
- Increased pain in the right lower quadrant upon coughing is the **Dunphy sign**, honoring British-American physician Osborne Joby Dunphy (1898–1989).
- Rebound tenderness is also called a positive **Blumberg sign**, after German physician Jacob Moritz Blumberg (1873–1955).
- **The Cope psoas test**, also called the **psoas sign**, is elicited by passively extending the thigh as the patient lies on his side with knees extended, or having the

patient actively flex his thigh at the hip. The term was introduced by British surgeon Zachary Cope (1881–1974), author of *Cope's Early Diagnosis of the Acute Abdomen*, first published in 1921.

• A patient who grimaces as the examiner sweeps the index and middle finger from the xiphoid to the right iliac fossa is said to have a positive **Massouh sign**. The sign is the brainchild of English surgeon Farouk Massouh, currently practicing in the United Kingdom at Frimley Park Hospital in Surrey.

A State of Premature Madness

One of the earliest terms describing a mental disorder distinguished by disconnections with reality was **dementia praecox**, meaning "premature madness," used in 1891 by Czech psychiatrist Arnold Pick (1851–1924), eponymized today in **Pick disease**, or **frontotemporal dementia**. The "praecox" in the name served to distinguish it from the dementias associated with aging, such as **Alzheimer disease**. The term **dementia praecox** languished until popularized by German psychiatrist Emil Kraepelin (1856–1926) in his book *Compendium of Psychiatry: For the Use of Students and Physicians*.

Then in 1911, Swiss psychiatrist Eugen Bleuler (1857–1939) introduced the term **schizophrenia**, from Greek words *schizein*, meaning "to split," and *phren*, or "mind" (Fig. 8.8). Bleuler described the manifestations of the disease as the four A's: **a**ssociations (loose), **a**mbivalence, **a**utism, and **a**ffective disturbance [5].

Bleuler's contributions to medical authorisms did not end with schizophrenia. He also coined the words **ambivalence**, **schizoid**, and **autism**, the latter term from the Greek *autos–*, "self," and *–ismos*, "state of." Thus, Bleuler's word **autism** describes a state of morbid self-absorption.

The Disease Resembling Flesh

An inflammatory disease of unknown origin, **sarcoidosis**, or simply **sarcoid**, can affect virtually any organ of the body. Although geographically widespread, it is especially common in persons of Scandinavian descent.

The disease was first described in 1877 by English dermatologist Jonathan Hutchinson (1828–1913), who told of a skin rash with raised erythematous lesions on the face and upper extremities. Hutchinson is remembered today for **Hutchinson teeth** (in congenital syphilis) (Fig. 8.9), **Hutchinson pupil** (seen with an intracranial mass lesion), and **Hutchinson sign** (vesicles on the tip of the nose that may herald the onset of herpes zoster ophthalmicus). But Hutchinson failed to give the newly recognized skin disease he described a name.

Sarcoidosis was first named in 1889 by Norwegian dermatologist Caesar Peter Møller Boeck (1845–1917), based on Greek *sarx*, meaning "flesh," and *eidos*,

Fig. 8.8 Eugen Bleuler.
Source: Zolliker Jahrheft
2011. Public Domain.
https://commons.
wikimedia.org/wiki/
File:Bleuler_Eugen.JPG

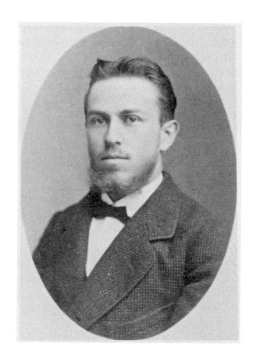

Fig. 8.9 Hutchinson teeth
resulting from congenital
syphilis. The permanent
incisor teeth are narrow
and notched. Note the
notched edges and
"screwdriver" shape of the
central incisors. Author:
CDC/Susan Lindsley.
Public Domain. https://
commons.wikimedia.org/
wiki/File:Hutchinson_
teeth_congenital_syphilis_
PHIL_2385_rsh.jpg

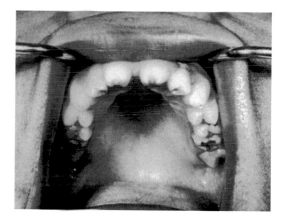

"resemblance." Others wrote of the disease, including French dermatologist Ernest Henri Besnier (1831–1909) and Swedish dermatologist Jörgen Nilsen Schaumann (1879–1953). In my research I came across the term **Besnier–Boeck–Schaumann disease**. But in most instances, the naming credit goes to Boeck, we sometimes call the disease **Boeck sarcoid**, and today the names of Besnier and Schaumann are seldom recalled in connection with **sarcoidosis**.

Perry, writing in 1949 (p. 83), opines of the word **sarcoid**, "In the present state of our ignorance, this is perhaps as good a name as any for this disease." Have we come much further in more than a half-century?

Dr. Röntgen's Mysterious Ray

Superman has **X-ray** vision, as did, slightly earlier, fictional heroine Olga Mesmer in a 1937–1938 comic strip. The word **X-radiation** was authored by German physicist Wilhelm Röntgen (1845–1922), after recognizing the phenomenon of electromagnetic radiation and sensing its potential.

In December 1895, Röntgen created the now-famous first medical X-ray of his wife's hand (Fig. 8.10). The "X" in the words X-radiation and X-ray was used by Röntgen to indicate that the nature of the rays was not understood. The existence of these almost-magical rays caught the public's imagination, sparking fear that unscrupulous persons might peer through clothing; to combat this danger, a London firm began to market "X-ray proof" undergarments.

A few years later, on the suggestion of Swiss physiologist Albert von Kölliker (1817–1905), the formal name was changed from X-rays to **Röntgen rays** (Garrison, p. 46). The English-speaking world came to know the phenomenon as **Roentgen rays**.

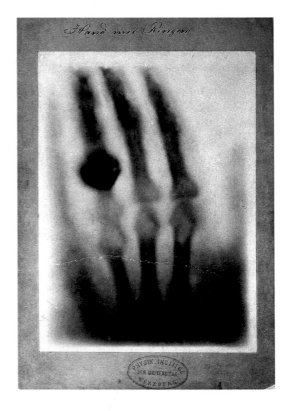

Fig. 8.10 Radiograph of hand by Wilhelm Roentgen, probably the hand of Frau Roentgen with a ring. Source: Wellcome Images. Public Domain. https://commons. wikimedia.org/wiki/ File:Radiograph_of_hand_ by_W.K._Roentgen_ Wellcome_L0000622EB. jpg

Radium, Polonium, and Curies

Three years after Roentgen imaged his wife's hand, Polish physicist Marie Curie (1867–1934) and her husband, French physicist Pierre Curie (1895–1906), working in Paris, discovered an element they named **polonium**, a term chosen to recognize Marie's native land, Poland. Later that same year, they described the existence of another element; they named this substance **radium**, from the Latin word *radius*, or "ray," based on the material's property of emitting energy as rays. Also at this time, they created the term **radioactivity**.

The Curies received the 1903 Nobel Prize in Physics, making Marie the first female Nobel laureate. Pierre died in 1906, struck by a horse-drawn vehicle while crossing a street in Paris. In his honor (at Marie's insistence) we have the **curie,** a unit of radioactivity. Marie was awarded many honors, including another Nobel Prize, before her death in 1934 from aplastic anemia, perhaps related to the test tubes of radium she carried in the pocket of her lab coat. Following its discovery in 1944, the radioactive chemical element with the atomic number 96 was named **curium**, to honor Marie and Pierre Curie (Fig. 8.11).

Fig. 8.11 Nobel portrait of Marie Curie, ca. 1903. Public Domain. https:// commons.wikimedia.org/ wiki/File:Marie-Curie-Nobel-portrait-600.jpg

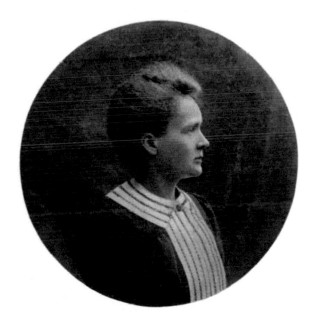

Sorry About the Mediterranean Jellyfish

In the early twentieth century, it seems that the royal family and guests of Monaco suffered jellyfish stings while swimming in the Mediterranean Sea. Could someone help these poor souls? Knowing of the work on immunity by Louis Pasteur and Robert Koch, French physiologist Charles Robert Richet (1850–1935) set out to find the answer.

Richet attempted to induce immunity in a dog by injecting the animal with small amounts of jellyfish venom. When, later, the dog was given a second injection of the venom, it became gravely ill instead of exhibiting immunity. Similar experiments in various animals yielded similar results, including some deaths. Although Richet could not explain what his findings meant, in 1902, he did name the phenomenon **anaphylaxis**, from Greek *ana–*, meaning "backward," and *phylaxis*, "protection," to describe the exaggerated response he had observed [6].

The Magic Bullet and Chemotherapy

German biochemist Paul Ehrlich (1854–1915) gave us two terms used today (Fig. 8.12). The first was **magic bullet**, a bit of a slang term for a drug that strikes a disease target without doing damage to the body. Ehrlich borrowed the term from German folktales of projectiles with astonishing accuracy, and he set out to find the magic bullet that might cure one of the scourges of his day—syphilis.

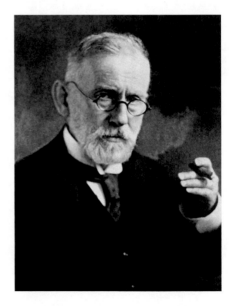

Fig. 8.12 Paul Ehrlich, ca. 1905–1910. Source: KRUIF, Paul de. *Mikrobenjäger*. Orell Füssli, Zürich, 1927. Public Domain. https://commons.wikimedia.org/wiki/File:Paul_Ehrlich_(1926-27_Microbe_Hunters).jpg

Ehrlich used a method still in vogue today. He diligently tested one compound after another until he found one that worked. Success came with the 606th compound tested, an organoarsenical drug first dubbed **compound 606**, and then **arsphenamine**, which was marketed in 1910 under the proprietary name **Salvarsan**. The word **Salvarsan** came from Latin *salvare*, meaning "to save," and arsphenamine was based on the German *Arsenik* or arsenic. The drug was intended to be the salvation of humankind—with arsenic as the active agent.

Salvarsan, safer and more effective than the previous antisyphilitic, mercury, enjoyed wide use until replaced by the somewhat more soluble compound **neoarsphenamine** (**Neosalvarsan**), the name constructed by adding Greek *neo–*, "new," to **Salvarsan**. This may make **Neosalvarsan** unique as a five-syllable medical word with origins in Greek, Latin, and German.

To describe this type of medication use, Ehrlich coined another term, **chemotherapy**, used today more in connection with anticancer drugs than for antimicrobials.

Being Dull and Worse

American psychologist Henry H. Goddard (1866–1957) gave medicine a new word, **moron**, from the Greek *moros*, meaning "dull," to describe persons with an intelligence quotient (IQ) between 51 and 70 (Forsyth, p. 186). In fact, being a moron was superior to being an **imbecile**, from Latin *imbecillus*, or "feeble", with an IQ of 26–50, or an **idiot**, from Greek *idiotes*, meaning "an unskilled person," with an IQ of zero to 25.

Moron was the name of a dim-witted character in Molière's play *La Princesses d'Elide*, written in the seventeenth century. Perhaps this fictional character came to mind as the American Psychological Association voted approval of the word in 1910, making moron one of the few words ever voted into the English language (Hendrickson, p. 234), and perhaps the even fewer medical words ever voted into existence. (The **curie**, described above, may be another.)

All these words—moron, imbecile, idiot, and feebleminded—are no longer used by psychologists or physicians, but remain as hateful epithets in the popular vocabulary.

No Thirteenth Floor in My Hotel

A morbid fear of the number "13" is called **triskaidekaphobia**. Ciardi (p. 392) describes that word as a whimsical British university invention of uncertain dating. Triskaidekaphobia comes from Greek *treiskaideka*, "thirteen," plus *phobia*, "fear." The word was first used in print by American psychiatrist Isador Coriat (1875–1943) in his 1910 book *Abnormal Psychology* [7].

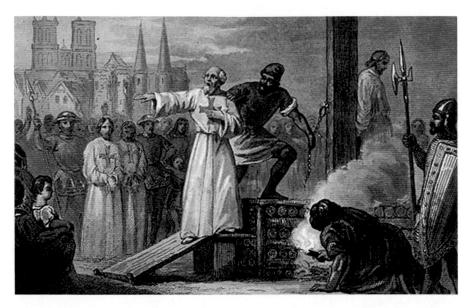

Fig. 8.13 Jacques de Molay saying that he is innocent. Author: Ignote. Public Domain. https://commons.wikimedia.org/wiki/File:Jacques_de_Molay_innocent.jpg

What is the source of triskaidekaphobia? The thirteenth law of the Babylonian Code of Hammurabi, dating to the eighteenth century BCE, is believed by some to be absent. Judas, the disciple who betrayed Jesus, was the thirteenth to sit at the last supper table. Viking tradition held that if thirteen persons met, one would die within the year. And Jacques de Molay and the Knights Templar were arrested by French King Philip IV on October 13, 1307, which also happened to be a Friday (Fig. 8.13). Perhaps this incident contributed to the superstition, **paraskevidekatriaphobia**, the fear of Friday the thirteenth.

And isn't it just a little spooky that as I sought images for this chapter, the figure that ended up illustrating fear of the number thirteen would be the thirteenth figure in the chapter? I did not plan this.

Discovering is Different than Naming

While studying canine liver cells in 1916, medical student Jay McLean, working in the laboratory of American physiologist William Henry Howell (1860–1945) at Johns Hopkins University, first isolated the **heparin**. McLean may have discovered the drug, but naming rights went to Howell, who coined the word **heparin**, from the Greek *hepar*, or "liver," referring to the original source of the anticoagulant.

Howell went on to become dean of the medical school from 1899 to 1901 (Fig. 8.14). In 1959, McLean described his discovery of heparin and how he had to convince a skeptical Howell that he had found what he called a "natural anticoagulant" [8].

Fig. 8.14 William Henry
Howell, 1911. Author:
Cecilia Beaux. Public
Domain. https://commons.
wikimedia.org/wiki/
File:William_Henry_
Howell_(painting,_1911).
jpg

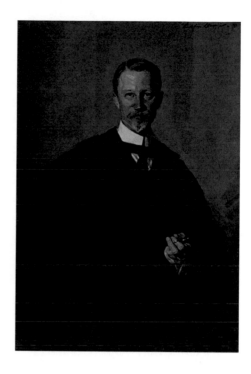

About Your Breath

In Chap. 7, I told the story of Joseph Lister and Listerine. One of the chief claims of the early purveyors of Listerine is that it cured **halitosis**—bad breath. George Lambert, son of Listerine founder Jordan Wheat Lambert, invented the word halitosis in 1921. The word combines Latin *halitus*, meaning "breath," with the Greek suffix *–osis*, medically indicating a "state of disease." Might this have been a word—and a disease—concocted to sell a mouthwash?

Medicine's Longest Word

What is the name of the type of pneumoconiosis cause by inhalation of minute particles of silica volcanic dust? The answer, **pneumonoultramicroscopicsilicovolcanoconiosis,** was not the creation of a physician or scientist. The 45-letter word was the invention of Everett M. Smith, president of the National Puzzlers' League. The term, which just might be a tongue-in-cheek invention, like attempting an unconventional *Guinness Book of World Records* feat, was first in print in 1935 in the *New York Herald Tribune* and then legitimized in the *Merriam Webster New International Dictionary*, second edition, published in 1939.

Naming the Early Wonder Drugs

The first antimicrobial drug proven to be effective against *Mycobacterium tuberculosis* was **streptomycin**, isolated in 1943 by then-graduate student Albert Schatz (1922–2005), working in the laboratory of American microbiologist Selman Waksman (1888–1973) in the Department of Soil Microbiology at Rutgers University. The 1944 paper announcing the discovery, with Schatz as first author, begins by describing "A new antibacterial substance, designated as streptomycin" [9].

The agent, like many antimicrobials to follow, came from microorganisms in the soil. Streptomycin was isolated from the soil-based bacterium *Streptomyces griseus*, and I think we can reasonably credit the word streptomycin to Schatz and assume that the "strepto" part of the word came from the name of the *Streptomyces* bacterium source.

There is less ambiguity about the author of the word **antibiotic**, meaning "against living things." This is credited to the senior scientist in the laboratory and terminal author on the paper, Selman Waksman. The epitaph on Waksman's gravestone reads: "Out of the earth shall come thy salvation" (Li, p. 66).

Not Everyone Favors a New Medical Word

Most authorisms have a single parent; a few have two. In 1954, Somerset Waters (1882–1970), travel consultant to US President Eisenhower, and American physician B. H. Kean (1912–1993) created the Travelers Health Institute, with the goal of reducing the incidence of traveler's diarrhea. The institute needed a letterhead and perhaps a catchy new name. What should it be? There was *pediatrics* for children and *geriatrics* for the elderly. A logical name for their endeavor was **emporiatrics**, from the Greek *emporos*, meaning "traveler."

Kean wrote, "I hated it. It reminded me of 'emporium,' the entrepreneurial euphemism for the musty, depressing corner dry-goods store ubiquitous in the Midwest of my youth—wholly inappropriate for an international organization of style and sophistication." But Waters persisted, and today **emporiatrics** is a recognized medical subspecialty involved in the health care of travelers. According to Kean: "Waters was the genius, but within medical circles at least, I usually get the credit" [10].

Gomer

Most physicians know the word **gomer**. If asked, they would probably attribute it to pseudonymous author Samuel Shem, who gave us the satirical novel *The House of God* (1978), about the hospital-based training of a group of medical interns. In

Shem's book gomer is actually an acronym for the phrase "Get Outta My Emergency Room!" It is intended to describe "a human being who has lost—often through aging—what goes into being a human being" [11]. In the medical setting—actually, in any setting—gomer is clearly, like the word moron, derogatory and tasteless. But maybe the word predates Shem.

There are several persons named Gomer in the Bible: In Genesis (10:2,3) Gomer is the eldest son of Japheth. In the Book of Hosea, the allegedly promiscuous wife of the prophet Hosea was named Gomer. Gomer Pyle was the character name of the country bumpkin, and later, US Marine in the television series *The Andy Griffith Show* (1960–1968) and *Gomer Pyle, USMC* (1964–1969). So was Shem's 1978 acronymic creation of gomer actually a **backronym**, where the word comes first and then initial letters are found to match the word, a device employed in naming many research studies?

Neither Diagnosed nor Cured

The term **heartsink patient** is probably used more often in Britain than in the United States, but the phenomenon knows no geographic boundaries. Simply stated, a heartsink patient is one whose name on the daily schedule makes the physician's heart sink. There can be many reasons for this emotion: The patient may be chronically late, demanding, clinging, or excessively talkative. The patient may be a "frequent flier," to use an American slang term, or simply one who presents repeatedly with obscure symptoms that can be neither diagnosed nor cured.

The term **heartsink patient** is attributed to Irish general practitioner Thomas C. O'Dowd, whose 1988 paper described five years of experience with these patients. The author writes: "While heartsink patients often have serious medical problems, they are a disparate group of individuals whose only common thread seems to be the distress they cause their doctor and the practice. Heartsink as a phenomenon has features that are unique to general practice" [12].

Diabetic and Overweight

What took us so long? For years we have recognized that obesity and diabetes often occur in the same patients and not by chance. Obesity is a risk factor for diabetes, and weight control is an important aspect of antidiabetic therapy.

Yet, it was not until 2005 that we saw the two disorders linked in a neologism. The word **diabesity** was created by American endocrinologist Francine Kaufman and introduced in her book titled *Diabesity: The Obesity-Diabetes Epidemic That Threatens America—And What We Must Do To Stop It* [13].

Into the Record, Over and Over

We have the **fascinoma**, an obscure finding that evokes a great deal of clinical interest. There is the **incidentaloma**, an unexpected finding on laboratory screening or imaging that may send the patient on a Ulysses syndrome odyssey, described in Chap. 2. There is even the **cheerioma**, a somewhat etymologically confusing term, relating to a patient with a malignant, aggressive tumor. The identities of the authors of these three slang terms are lost in history. But there are two more of these *–oma* authorisms, the creator of which is well known.

In 2008, American physician Abraham Verghese gave us two new authorisms in a single paper (Fig. 8.15). The first was **iPatient**, described in Chap. 1. The second, a product of our electronic medical records in which a chart note—accurate or not—can be cut and pasted into the record day after day, is the word **chartoma**. Verghese describes chartomas as "disease labels immortalized by being cut and pasted into every note so that by sheer repetition, a whiff of tricuspid insufficiency turns into a raging torrent" [14].

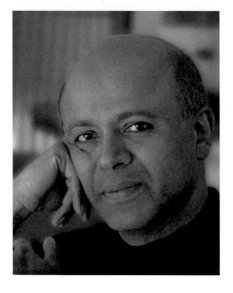

Fig. 8.15 Abraham Verghese. Author: Mcjudy. Creative Commons. https://commons.wikimedia.org/wiki/File:Verghese,_Abraham,_blurred_2.jpg

References

1. Koestler, A. The sleepwalkers: a history of man's changing vision of the Universe. London: Penguin Books; 1972, pp. 26-42.
2. Harding SE. Everything old is new again. J Gerontol A Biol Sci Med Sci. 2009; 64A:149.
3. Kovner SG. Erasistratus. Available at: http://encyclopedia2.thefreedictionary.com/Erasistratus+of+Ceos
4. Bergman NA. Michael Faraday and his contribution to anesthesia. Anesthesiology. 1992;77:812.
5. Rosen H. A guide to clinical psychiatry, 2nd ed. Miami FL: Mnemosyne Publishing; 1978.
6. Bollett AJ. Medical history in medical terminology. Res Staff Phys. 1999;45(9):60.
7. Coriat I. Abnormal psychology. New York: Moffat, Yard, and Co.; 1910, p. 319.
8. McLean J. The discovery of heparin. Circulation. 1959;19:75.
9. Schatz A, Bugle E, Waksman SA. Streptomycin, a substance exhibiting antibiotic activity against gram-positive and gram-negative bacteria. Exp Biol Med (Maywood). 1944;55:66.
10. Kean BH. Emporiatrics. Atlantic magazine. 1990;266(6):19. Available at: http://www.dountoothers.org/odd41807.htm.
11. Shem S. The house of God. New York, Dell, 1978.
12. O'Dowd TC. Five years of heartsink patients. BMJ. 1998;297:528.
13. Kaufman F. Diabesity: The obesity-diabetes epidemic that threatens America—and what we must do to stop it. New York: Bantam; 2005.
14. Verghese A. Culture shock—patient as icon, icon as patient. N Engl J Med. 2008;359;2748.

Chapter 9
Medical Words with Intriguing Origins

Some medical words, such as **ptosis** and **tibia**, come to us directly from ancient Greek or Latin. Other terms we use link together prefixes, roots, and suffixes from these sources to create words such as **antibiotic** and **cardiology**. But the sources of some of our current medical words are less obvious. Some have intriguing backstories, and others are based on historical misperceptions.

This chapter tells about the confusion between the diaphragm and the mind, preserved in our word **phrenic**, what the ancients believed was the cause of **influenza**, how the word **placebo** arose from a verse in the Bible, the medical word created in a Boston tavern, and the tale behind the "unnamed" artery. We explore terms used in anatomy, diseases, microorganisms, and drug names, as well as some esoteric medical words, a few health-related euphemisms, and the rise of the use of acronyms in medicine.

From Mind to Diaphragm

In classical Greek, the word *phren* meant "mind." From this we have the word **schizophrenic**, "split mind," and **phrenology**, "study of the mind," which is actually a pseudoscience involved with study of the human skull (Fig. 9.1). Even the modern words **frenzy**, **frenetic**, and **frantic** trace their origins to the Greek word *phren*. Yet, the ancient Greeks noticed that a strong emotion could cause a tightening of the upper abdominal muscles, and they logically assumed this area to be the seat of emotions. Thus began the spurious connection between the mind and the **diaphragm**.

In *On the Sacred Disease*, Hippocrates (ca. 460–377 BCE) attempted to dispel the confusion, and eventually physicians and scientists placed the mind in its proper cranial location. But the linguistic misperception persisted, and today we have the **phrenic nerve** (yes, named for the "mind"), originating in the cervical spine and descending through the thorax on its journey to the diaphragm.

© Springer International Publishing AG 2017
R.B. Taylor, *The Amazing Language of Medicine*,
DOI 10.1007/978-3-319-50328-8_9

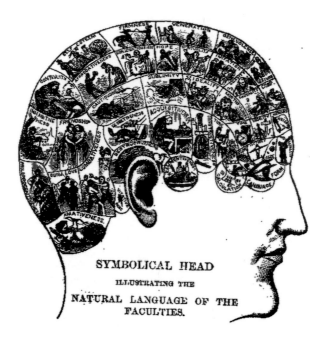

SYMBOLICAL HEAD
ILLUSTRATING THE
NATURAL LANGUAGE OF THE
FACULTIES.

Fig. 9.1 Phrenology chart from the nineteenth century. Source: Fowlers & Wells. Public Domain. https://commons.wikimedia.org/wiki/File:Phrenologychart.png

On the Influence of the Stars

In 1580, in his *History of Florence*, Italian historian Domenico Buoninsegni wrote of *influentia coeli*, or "celestial influence," to describe an **influenza** epidemic during 1357 (Garrison, p. 187). Ackerknecht (p. 74) tells of an 1173 flu epidemic in Italy, Germany, and England, two epidemics in the fourteenth century, and three in the fifteenth. With all the various waves of contagion sweeping across the known world during ancient times, the Middle Ages, and the Renaissance, it is no wonder that those living in fear of these diseases would attribute influenza to the gods and the stars.

In later years, some created names to blame others: Germans called influenza "the Russian pestilence," the Russians called it "the Chinese disease," and even the Italians came to use the term "the German disease." According to Garrison (p. 404), English surgeon John Huxham (1692–1768) was the first to use the word influenza in English, in his 1767 description of the "vernal catarrh" of 1743. We no longer subscribe to the notion of heavenly influence, although we still occasionally fix blame on others (**Hong Kong flu**) and even animals (**swine flu**).

From Under the Costal Cartilages

Under the costal cartilages lie the liver on the right and the spleen on the left. To these organs, the ancients attributed a number of disorders, such as *melancholia* ("black bile") from the liver, giving us our current word **melancholy**. Other words emerging from this misperception were **bilious, liverish**, and **splenetic**—descriptive terms no longer used in modern medicine.

Because various psychosomatic illnesses were ascribed to these organs housed under the lower ribs, a person with the unfounded belief that he or she was ill came to be called a **hypochondriac**, from the Greek prefix *hypo–*, "under," plus *khondros*, "cartilage." The condition came to be called **hypochondriasis** (Fig. 9.2). In the academic setting, it has been termed **medical student disease**.

Jamieson tells an anecdote about English physician Thomas Sydenham (1625–1689) who, at his wits' end with a hypochondriacal patient, sent him to consult with an esteemed physician in Scotland. The journey by stagecoach was taxing, and, at the end of his journey, the patient was furious to discover that the consultant physician was a fiction. As Jamieson states, "He returned to London full of rage, but cured of the complaint" [1].

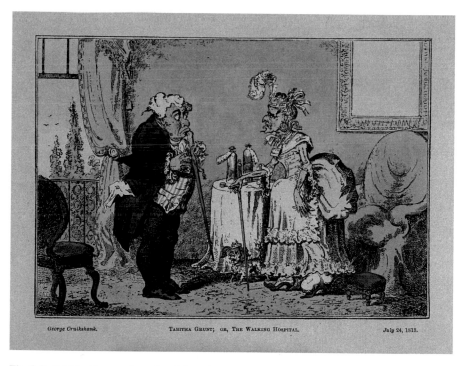

Fig. 9.2 Tabitha Grunt, a hypochondriac who appears to suffer from many illnesses, consulting a bemused looking doctor. Colored reproduction of an etching after G. Cruikshank, 1813. Source: Wellcome images. Public Domain. https://commons.wikimedia.org/wiki/File:Tabitha_Grunt_a_hypochondriac_who_appears_to_suffer_from_man_Wellcome_V0010980.jpg

Fornicate

The word describing the act of sexual intercourse, often with the connotation of sex between unmarried persons, **fornicate**, has an appropriately spicy origin. The word began with the Latin *fornix*, meaning "vault" or "arch." There is also a **vaginal fornix**, from the same Latin root, alluding to the shape of the superior portion of the vagina.

In ancient Rome, brothels were built at basement level, with vaulted ceilings. Enterprising ladies—the sex providers of their day—sometimes sought clients while standing under the arched entrances to their establishments. From this architectural feature, according to Ciardi (p. 137), early Christian writers created the term *fornicari*, referring to those who frequent brothels. In the sixteenth century, we added the female forms of the word: **fornicatrice**, **fornicatrix**, and **fornicatress**. Today, in polite company we often use the euphemism "intercourse" instead of **fornicate**.

Of Our Own Making

A **nostrum** is a medicine, generally one that is patented but which is considered not especially effective. The word comes from the Latin *noster*, meaning "our," and connotes that the remedy is "of our own making." As stated by Karlen, "ours does it, cures everything from pip to pimples. Some are outright fakes, some the work of earnest cultists; some represent a grain of medical truth inflated to baroque, all-encompassing systems" [2].

In 1870, a patient could buy *Mugwump Remedy*, a cure and preventive for all venereal diseases. *Kickapoo Indian Sagwa*, a blood, liver, and stomach renovator, was sold at medicine shows and was probably the inspiration for *Kickapoo Joy Juice* found in the *Li'l Abner* comic strip by Al Capp (1909–1979).

Some nostrums are still with us. One is *Lydia E. Pinkham's Vegetable Compound*, originally containing a whopping 18% ethanol, now marketed as *Lydia Pinkham Herbal Compound*, which contains dandelion, gentian, motherwort, pleurisy root, black cohosh, and Jamaican dogwood, but with only 10% ethanol (Fig. 9.3). The age of the nostrum has not ended. As English poet George Crabbe (1754–1832) wrote (Garrison, p. 384):

From the poor man's pay
The nostrum takes no trifling part away.

I Shall Be Pleasing

A medicine or procedure that can cause no harm but that provides no physical benefit to the patient is called a **placebo**. The word has Biblical origins.

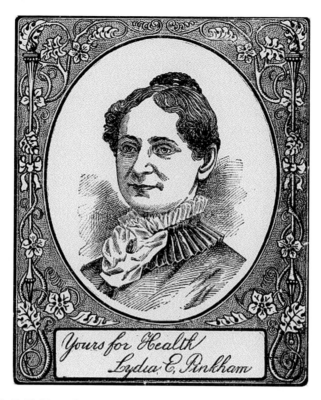

Fig. 9.3 Lydia E. Pinkham. Source: Dpbsmith. Public domain. https://commons.wikimedia.org/wiki/File:Lydiapinkham-007.png

The *Vulgate* is a Latin translation of the Bible, dating to the fourth century, that was adopted in the sixteenth century as the official version of the Catholic Church. In this version of the Bible, Psalm 114, verse 9 reads: "*Placebo Domino in regione vivorum.*" Translated, this sentence means, "I shall be pleasing unto the Lord in the Land of the Living." This phrasing was adopted as the first antiphon at Vespers at the Office of the Dead (Evans IH, 1970, p. 841).

As flatterers sang the *Placebo* in an effort to obtain benefits of some sort from the relatives of the dead, the term "to sing placebo" came to mean one who pleases in the sense of providing something that seemed to gratify without harming. The word formally entered the medical dictionary in 1811, when defined as "[any medicine] adapted more to please than benefit the patient" in *John Quincy's Lexicon Medicum*, edited by English physician Robert Hooper (1733–1835).

We now know that the placebo can have effects, both favorable and not. In any placebo-controlled drug study, some subjects receiving inert substances will develop adverse effects, such as nausea, headache, or fatigue. This is called the **nocebo effect**, from the Latin *nocebo*, "I shall harm."

Compassion for One with a Soul

Like *moron, idiot*, and *mongolism*, the word **cretin** is now dated, and preferred terms are **hypothyroidism** or **myxedema**. When it was part of our everyday medical vocabulary, cretin described a person who was mentally and physically handicapped because of a thyroid deficiency—whether congenital or acquired.

Even though no longer entered in our medical records, the word has a curious origin worth considering. The tale begins with Paracelsus (1493–1541), who recognized the connection between parents with goiters and offspring who were "feeble-minded" (to use another outdated term) with stunted growth (Haubrich, p. 55). Then in the eighteenth and nineteenth centuries, in the valleys of the mountains of Europe, observers noted a number of persons with deformed bodies and low intelligence, the result of a diet chronically deficient in iodine. They came to be called the *Cretins of the Alps* (Fig. 9.4).

The word cretin arose from the Old French *crétin*, coming from *Vulgar* Latin word *christianus*, to mean "a Christian." The word *cretin*, applied to these brutish creatures, was intended to be compassionate to one who has a God-given soul. Today the word cretin is more likely to be used in common parlance, and in a derogative manner, than in serious clinical conversation.

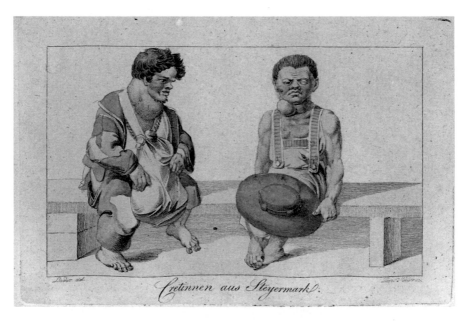

Fig. 9.4 Cretins, early nineteenth century. Source: Oesterreichs Tibur. Scanned by Hubertl. Public Domain. https://commons.wikimedia.org/wiki/File:Cretinnen_aus_Steiermark,_1819_gez._Loder,_gest._Leopold_Müller.jpg

Like a Bird Flapping its Wings

A tremor of the hand when the wrist is extended is called **asterixis**, also known as a **flapping tremor** or a **liver flap**. The word comes from the Greek prefix *a–*, or "not," and *sterixis*, "fixed position." The phenomenon has been likened to a bird flapping its wings. Asterixis is seen in various metabolic encephalopathies, notably with liver failure, as well as in patients with respiratory failure and Wilson disease.

According to Sapira (Orient, p. 581), the word asterixis was invented by American neurologist Joseph Michael Foley (1916–2012) in a Greek bar in Boston called *The Taverna*. Foley consulted Jesuit scholar Father Cardigan, who preferred the term **anisosterixis**, from *aniso–*, or "unequal," and *sterixis*. But asterixis was a better descriptor of the flapping tremor and was simply a shorter word.

Archery and Toxins

It might seem curious that the word **toxin**, meaning a "poisonous substance" comes from the Greek *toxon*, or "bow." When archers began to dip their arrowheads in poison, the poison arrows were called *toxikon pharmakon*. The apparent confusion between bow and arrow continued until 1545, when English author Roger Ascham (1515–1568) wrote a book titled *Toxophilus*, meaning "lover of the bow" (Shipley, p. 195). Eventually the Greek *toxikon* was Latinized to *toxicon*. Then in 1886, the word toxin came into use to designate something that can cause bodily harm. From the parent word toxin, we developed the terms **toxic, toxoid, toxicity,** and **antitoxin** (Perry, p. 96). We also have **neurotoxins, cytotoxins, mycotoxins,** and more.

The etymologic connection with bow and arrow endures in the term **toxophilite**, describing one who is fond of archery.

The Packsaddle Child

The word **bastard** may not be exactly a medical term, but I include it here because of its colorful origin. Although sometimes used as an insult, the word simply denotes a person born of parents not married to each other. There have been some noteworthy illegitimate children: The first Norman king of England, William the Conqueror (1028–1087), was also known as William the Bastard. American statesman Alexander Hamilton (1755–1804) was called by John Adams and Thomas Jefferson "the bastard brat of a Scots pedlar" (Rawson, p. 30).

Etymologically speaking, the word is fairly new. Bastard arose from a descriptive term, coming from the Old French, *fils de bast*, or "packsaddle child" (Fig. 9.5). Riders typically used the packsaddle, the *bast*, as a bed. Today we have several euphemisms used instead of bastard: love child, born on the wrong side of the blanket, and born out of wedlock.

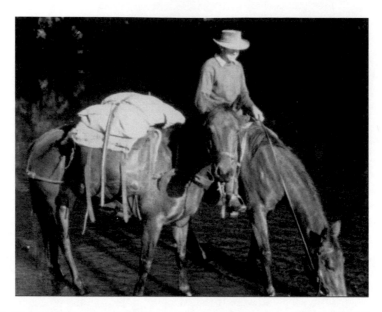

Fig. 9.5 The packhorse is carrying an army style packsaddle, with pack bags and bedding on top. Author: Matthew Goodwin. Public Domain. https://commons.wikimedia.org/wiki/File:Pack_Horse_2.jpg

The Place of the Skull

The **calvarium** is the skullcap, the skull minus the facial bones and mandible. The word comes from the Latin *calvaria,* "skull", which in turn comes from *calvus*, meaning "bald." **Cranium** is derived from the Greek *kraniou topos*, which was how the Greeks translated the Aramaic word *gulgulta*, or "place of the skull." The intriguing connection is the name of the site of Christ's crucifixion hill outside the walls of Jerusalem. Even today, the contour of the hill suggests a skull. The location was called Golgotha, "skull hill" in Aramaic, and later Calvary in Latin (Gershen, p. 6).

Here are some more anatomical sites with interesting names.

The Measure of the Elbow

The **cubital fossa**, sometimes termed the **elbow pit**, is the anterior aspect of the elbow, containing various nerves, tendons, arteries, and veins. Many clinicians prefer the term **antecubital fossa**, meaning "in front of the elbow," which seems a little more precise.

The word root **cubit** is from Latin *cubitum*, or "elbow." But physicians do not have the only claim on the **cubit**, which is also an ancient unit of measure, the distance from the elbow to the tip of the middle finger, about 18–20 in. in today's reckoning. Because patrician Romans preferred to eat while reclining, using their

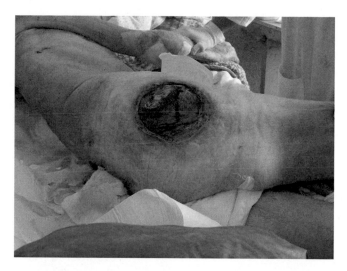

Fig. 9.6 Stage 4 decubitus ulcer displaying the Gluteus medius muscle attached to the crest of the ilium. Author: Bobjalindo. Creative Commons. https://commons.wikimedia.org/wiki/File:Imagen_Bob_108.jpg

elbows for support, the cubit (elbow) became linked with the supine position, giving us the words **incubate**, "to lie on," and **decubitus**, "to lie down." Today the latter term is often associated with a pressure sore, described clinically as a **decubitus ulcer** (Fig. 9.6).

The Humorous Humerus

The long bone of the arm, extending from the shoulder to the elbow, is the **humerus**, adapting the Latin word with the same spelling. So far this is ho-hum etymology. But there is a "humorous" (sorry about that) twist. The ulnar nerve runs by the medial condyle of the humerus, and when struck, the person experiences sudden, lancinating pain. According to Hendrickson (p. 170): "Nothing is very funny about this—it inspires cursing rather than laughter—but Barham or some other punster before him probably saw the pun humorous in the humerus bone and dubbed it the **funny bone** [or **crazy bone**, if you prefer], adding one the few puns that have become words to the language."

The No-Name Artery

In the second century CE, Greek physician Claudius Galen (129–200) was surgeon to the gladiators, who made a business of cutting up one another in the Roman Forum. He was physician to three emperors and he was the one first to map the arteries of the aortic arch.

But, whoops. He failed to name one of the major branches coming from the aortic arch. The oversight was discovered more than a millennium later, as the world emerged from the medieval suspension of scientific thought, by Italian anatomist Andreas Vesalius (1514–1564) in Padua, Italy. He named it the **innominate artery**, the "no name" artery, a scientific term still used today.

Not to have a good term be underutilized, we also have the **innominate bone**, also known as the hipbone, and the **innominate vein**, also called the **brachiocephalic vein**.

Philtrum

Also called the medial cleft, the **philtrum** is a midline vertical depression above the upper lip. In his book *Gabriel's Palace: Jewish Mystical Tales* [3], American scholar Howard Schwartz tells that Lailah, the guardian angel who watches over all our days and who, in the end, will lead us to the *world to come*, touches an infant's upper lip before birth, creating the depression (Fig. 9.7).

Functionally, the **philtrum** may serve to carry moisture from the mouth to keep the nose wet. The word comes from the Greek *philtron*, meaning "love potion" or "charm." Dirckx (p. 61) observes: "Those who profess not to see the connection have been at their books too long."

A Disease Your Friends Diagnose

According to medical scholar Sir William Osler (1848–1919), **jaundice** is a disease that your friends diagnose. The word comes from the Old French *jaune*, meaning "yellow." To describe the yellow-green skin caused by bile pigments in the blood,

Fig. 9.7 Philtrum of an infant. Photo by VanessaQ. Creative Commons. https://commons.wikimedia.org/wiki/File:Surprised.jpg

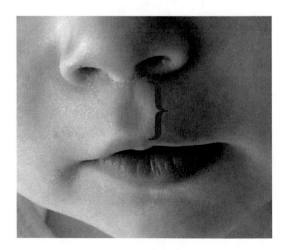

we often use the term **icterus**, from the Greek *icterus*, which was the name of a yellow-feathered bird that, when sighted, could cure jaundice. Today we have the genus *Icterus* of the blackbird family, of which the Baltimore oriole (*Icterus galbula*) has a yellow breast. But, of course, avian sighting cures notwithstanding, jaundice is clinical sign and not a disease.

Jaundice indicates liver disease, often caused by **cirrhosis**. Jamieson tells that French physician René Laënnec (1781–1826) named the disease in 1826, drawing upon the Greek word *kirrhos*, meaning "tawny, yellow." Today Laënnec is more remembered for his invention of the stethoscope than for his neologism, cirrhosis [4].

Hippocrates and the Fox

At this point in the chapter, I turn our attention to some diseases with unlikely etymologies. Consider **alopecia**, the scientific term for baldness. The word comes the Greek *alopecia*, meaning "loss of fur" or "fox mange." An even earlier Greek word was *alopex*, or "fox." What is the connection between baldness and the fox? There are two possibilities. The first is that the fox sheds its fur twice a year and appears hairless after the shedding. The second is that foxes afflicted with the mange lose hair.

Clinically we encounter **alopecia areata** (patchy hair loss) (Fig. 9.8) and **alopecia totalis** (total hair loss), but the most common type of baldness is **androgenic alopecia**, or male pattern baldness. Hippocrates had male pattern baldness, and one Internet source, undoubtedly reliable, tells that Hippocrates treated his androgenic alopecia by applying a "concoction of opium, horseradish, pigeon droppings, beetroot, and spices" [5]. Even the father of medicine, it seems, was not immune to the promises of the nostrums of his time.

A Synonym for Syphilis

In times, a few generations ago, when **syphilis** was more prevalent than today, physicians often used the words **lues** and **luetic**. In Latin, the word *lues* refers to an "infection" or "contagious disease." The use of the word became narrowed to mean syphilis following the 1835 work of French physician Philippe Ricord (1799–1889), whose research involving Parisian prostitutes established that syphilis and **gonorrhea** were different diseases (Haubrich, p. 128). In his honor, the initial skin lesion of lues has been called the **Ricord chancre**.

Linguistic purists will note that the word lues is singular, and there is no word "lue."

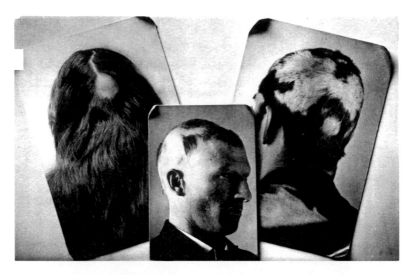

Fig. 9.8 Alopecia areata. Author: George Henry Fox. Public Domain. https://commons.wikime-dia.org/wiki/File:Alopecia_areata.jpg

A Curious Numerical Name for an Illness

In Chap. 6, I told of the **slapped cheek syndrome**, a febrile cold-like childhood ill-ness characterized by a bright red rash on the cheeks. German physician Anton Tschamer was first to use the term "slapped cheeks" in 1889 [6]. The disease is formally designated as **erythema infectiosum**, but is also known as **fifth disease**, a term coined by Cheinisse in 1905 [7].

A numerical designation is a curious name for an illness. Who can name the four illnesses preceding fifth disease? And is there a sixth disease? Here they are:

1. Measles
2. Scarlet fever
3. Rubella
4. Duke disease, never associated with an organism, and a term not used today
5. Fifth disease
6. And, yes, there is a sixth disease: roseola, also known as exanthem subitum

Can You Die of a Broken Heart?

Stress cardiomyopathy may present with dyspnea, chest pain, palpitations, and diaphoresis. There may be hypotension, heart failure, or even shock. The disorder is caused by the action of stress-related hormones, such as adrenaline, on heart cells. It is caused by physical or emotional stress, the latter perhaps triggered by fear,

Fig. 9.9 Left ventriculography during systole showing apical ballooning akinesis with basal hyperkinesis in a characteristic takotsubo ventricle. Author: Tara C Gangadhar, Elisabeth Von der Lohe, Stephen G Sawada and Paul R Helft. Creative Commons. https://commons.wikimedia.org/wiki/File:Takotsubo_ventriculography.gif

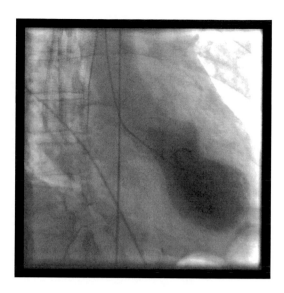

anger, or grief, such as loss of a loved one. Even a pleasurable surprise can trigger the syndrome.

I mention stress cardiomyopathy here because it has two fascinating nicknames. One is the **broken heart syndrome**, so-called because of its association with loss-related emotional stress. The other name sometimes heard is **takotsubo syndrome**. The disease, first described in Japan, causes a ballooning of the heart's left ventricle that resembles the narrow-necked, round bottom *tako-tsubo* pot, used by the Japanese to trap octopi (Fig. 9.9).

About Removing Feathers and More

My online medical dictionary lists an uncommon clinical entity: **ecdysiasm**. The term, describing an abnormal tendency to disrobe, comes from the Greek *ekdyein*, "to strip off one's clothes."

Although the term ecdysiasm is unlikely to be heard in everyday clinical conversation, there is a charming story behind the word **ecdysiast**, describing one who removes clothes. It seems that in 1940, American writer H. L. Mencken (1880–1956) received an unusual request. Miss Georgia Southern, whose profession was disrobing to music in front of an audience, was searching for a more dignified term for her work than "strip-teasing." Menken recalled the term *ecdysis*, the scientific name for molting—shedding feathers or skin. He proposed to Ms. Southern the term ecdysiast, still heard today in more sophisticated discourse as a euphemism for one whose profession is stripping (Ransom, p. 84).

Stirring the Pot

Here I tell the name of a syndrome you have probably never heard about, but have often encountered. Now you will be able to label the disorder—the **Kochleffel syndrome**—and know the origin of the term.

The first, and perhaps only, report of the disease is by Klein and Kaplinsky in Israel. The authors identify the word roots as German *Koch*, "cook," and *Loeffel*, "spoon." The syndrome is manifested by being a busybody who stirs things and people up. "Its most striking form is remarkably abrupt in onset and transforms the most charming person instantly into an excited, churning, and brewing creature with agitated behavior and delusions that curiously mimic those of paranoia." The authors theorize that the name of the disorder can be traced to Doctor Logophilus Acerbus von Kochloeffel (1780–1812), who, during Napoleon's invasion of Russia, was able to "cook up" entire meals for many from mere scraps of food. Kochloeffel's report of his achievements was rejected by journal editors, and he died "brokenhearted as a result of having made a mountain out of a molehill and having contracted the illness himself" [8].

Q is for Query, or Queensland

Only one disease is known by a single letter: **Q fever**. The disease, caused by *Coxiella burnetii*, causes flu-like symptoms of fever, headache, malaise, and muscle aches. Both humans and animals can be infected. How did it get the name Q fever?

The first description was by Australian pathologist Edward Holbrook Derrick (1898–1976), compiled after studying the disease in slaughterhouse workers in Queensland, Australia [9]. According to Dirckx (p. 74), the disease was named with the letter "Q" for query, indicating that the causative agent was unknown at the time of the original report. The term Q fever has endured in spite of other suggested names, including **abattoir fever** and **Queensland rickettsial fever**. Later, when the cause became known, the "Q" was retained, perhaps because of its original discovery in Queensland (Fig. 9.10).

It is just as well that Queensland rickettsial fever was not chosen as the name of the disease, because we now know that the *Coxiella burnetii* bacterium is morphologically similar to, but is not, when it comes to taxonomy, a member of the *Rickettsia* genus of bacteria.

Paregoric Politics

Turning from diseases to the drugs used to treat them, I will begin with a remedy that has been with us, in various modifications, for three centuries. The Greek sources of our word **paregoric** are *para–*, "beside," and *agoreuein*, "to speak in

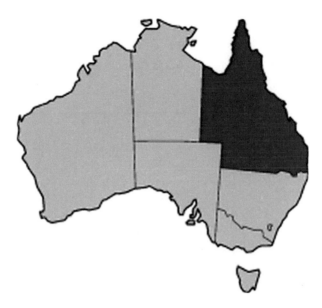

Fig. 9.10 Queensland in Australia. Author: Tim Starling. Creative Commons. https://commons. wikimedia.org/wiki/File:QLD_in_Australia_map.png

public." Think of the *agora*, "public space" as in **agoraphobia**. Thus, considering the original Greek roots, the literal sense of the word **paregoric** is "not engaged in politics." The connotation of the Greek word *paregorikos* is "soothing, inducing peace." The connection seems to be this: The Greeks wisely associated serenity with not being enmeshed in political discourse (Ciardi, p. 293).

Paregoric, describing camphorated **tincture of opium**, was first concocted—and named—by Dutch chemistry professor Jakob Le Mort (1650–1718). Le Mort's original formula included opium and wine, plus honey, licorice, flowers of Benjamin, salt of tartar, and oil of aniseed. It was marketed as *Elixir Asthmaticum* in 1721.

Over the years various odd substances were added to opium and alcohol, and the mixture changed often. A current formula for **paregoric U.S.P.** is benzoic acid, anise oil, anhydrous morphine, and 45 % alcohol. Its use today is to quell severe diarrhea. Lerner, however, has characterized paregoric as a "needless complex pharmacopeial mixture" [10]. Lerner makes no comment about being or not being engaged in political disagreements.

Like a Hero

Among the drugs used to relieve pain, **heroin** is still one of our most potent analgesics, despite the misery that misuse has caused over the years. The story begins in a laboratory at St. Mary's Hospital in London. It was here that in 1874, British chemist Charles Romley Alder Wright (1844–1894) first synthesized diacetylmorphine.

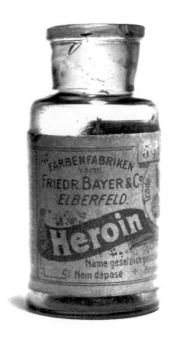

Wright tested the drug by feeding it to his dogs; the animals promptly spat it out, showing greater wisdom than humans who use the drug illicitly today.

Two decades later, German chemist Felix Hoffmann (1868–1946) at the Bayer AG pharmaceutical company used Wright's laboratory technique to "rediscover" diacetylmorphine, which Bayer scientists believed would prove to be a best-selling nonaddictive analgesic.

Another Bayer chemist, Heinrich Dreser (1860–1924), tested the drug on Bayer employees who volunteered for the project and on himself. The workers who took the drug found that it gave them a sense of euphoria, of exhilaration, or of being invincible. They felt heroic. Dresser gave his drug the trade name **Heroin**, from the word "hero," and beginning in 1888, it was promoted as a safe antitussive and alternative to morphine for the relief of pain (Li, p. 163) (Fig. 9.11).

Heroin fulfilled its promise in the relief of pain, and remains one of our most effective analgesics, but the claims of safety proved to be unfounded. In 1913, Bayer ceased production of heroin.

Rifamycins

The original source of the antibiotic **rifampicin,** also called **rifampin**, was from a soil sample taken in 1957 near the town of St. Raphael on the French Riviera. From this sample, researchers at Lepitit Pharmaceuticals in Milan, Italy discovered a new soil bacterium, *Streptomyces mediterranei*, which yielded several compounds with antimicrobial potential.

A popular film at this time was the French crime thriller *Rififi*, released in 1955. The Italian researchers, inspired by this movie, named their group of newly discovered group of molecules **rifamycins**. From these, we now have, in addition to rifampicin and rifampin, **rifabutin** and **rifaximin** [11].

Isoniazid

Although the etymology of the word **isoniazid** may be pedestrian, the tale of the antituberculosis drug is a noteworthy example of scientific coincidence and corporate wisdom.

It was a clash of Titans that ended with compromise. In 1946, American pharmaceutical company E. R. Squibb and Sons set out to find a second antituberculosis drug; the first such drug, **streptomycin**, had been developed in 1943. Using mice as subjects, in 1951 the researchers discovered a compound—**isonicotinic acid hydrazide**—that could protect mice against previously lethal injections of tubercle bacilli. They named the new drug **nydrazid**, based on the name of the chemical, and it was off to market.

But wait. From Switzerland came news that pharmaceutical firm F. Hoffmann-La Roche had discovered the same drug, demonstrated its antituberculosis action at virtually the same time, and named the drug **isoniazid**, also cobbling together bits from the drug's chemical name. Who owned rights to the drug? To resolve the dilemma, the companies agreed to place dated research notes of both laboratories in a hat. The company whose notes were picked containing the earlier date (Hoffman-La Roche) received patent rights; the runner-up on research note dates (Squibb) was granted a royalty-free license to manufacture and sell the product.

As the saying goes, no good deed—or no wise act—goes unpunished. Upon applying for a patent, Hoffman-La Roche learned of a claim predating those of both compromising firms, and neither pharmaceutical company received the profits expected for their work (Bordley, Harvey, p. 160).

From a Messy Diaper in Munich

While studying the intestinal bacteria of newborns and infants in 1885, German pediatrician Theodor Escherich (1857–1911) discovered an organism he called *Bacterium coli commune*, a logical name for a bacterium found in the large intestine. But the name given by Escherich was not destined to be the final choice.

In 1889, the name of the bacterium was changed to *Bacillus escherichia*, honoring the discoverer. In 1895, it was renamed *Bacillus coli* by German botanist Walter

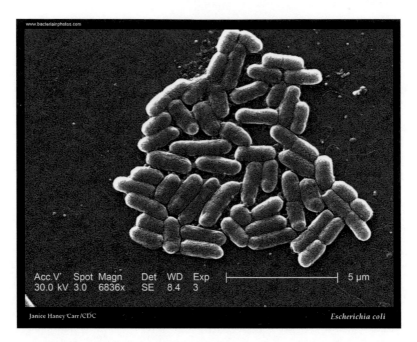

Fig. 9.12 Escherichia coli, strain, 157:H7. Author: Janice Haney Carr. Public Domain. https://commons.wikimedia.org/wiki/File:Escherichia_coli_electron_microscopy.jpg

Migula (1863–1938). Then in 1919, the organism received today's name, *Escherichia coli*, or *E. coli*, with the publication of the third edition of the *Manual of Tropical Medicine* (Fig. 9.12). This name seems likely to remain in the dictionary—until those capricious microbiologists decide to rename the organism again.

In the words of Morowitz: "Today's wonder bug entered human history in the messy diaper of a Munich infant, a truly modest start for the most widely chronicled organism in modern biology" [12].

Passing Through the Filter

In Latin, the word *virus* means "poison" or "slimy liquid." Later, in Middle English, **virus** came to mean "venom, as of a snake" (Maleska, p. 64). The word persisted in use as a general descriptor for a toxic substance. A 1702 description of Cleopatra's death describes her as succumbing to the "virus of an asp." In 1800, virus was vaguely used to refer to the cause of a disease: "the pustules contain a perfect smallpox virus" [13]. This was long before the discovery of the microorganisms we call virus today.

In 1885, French microbiologist Louis Pasteur (1822–1895) created the first rabies vaccine but could not identify a bacterial cause; he wondered about an organism too small to be seen under his microscope [14]. Then, in 1892, Russian botanist

Dmitri Ivanovsky (1864–1920) found that something that could pass through a filter could infect tobacco plants. Dutch microbiologist Martinus Beijerinck (1851–1931) showed in 1898 that whatever was passing through the filters was much smaller than bacteria; he is the one who began the use of the term virus to describe whatever it was that they had found. It was not until the invention of the electron microscope in the 1930s that scientists had their first look at viruses. The first human disease identified as caused by a virus was yellow fever (Sebastian, p. 750).

Linguistic Oddities

English, and especially the English-language medical dictionary, provides a panoply of words—offering a much richer selection than found in any other language. For example, the word **pandiculation** means to stretch the arms and torso, as when yawning. The word comes from Latin *pandiculari*, "to stretch oneself." Here are a few others you may not hear often, but they are there for use when needed.

Swearing to relieve stress or pain is **lalochezia**. The word comes from Ancient Greek *lalia*, meaning "speech," and *khezo*, "to defecate." This is related to the word **coprolalia**, the involuntary use of profanity as a disease symptom, from the Greek word *kopros*, meaning "dung," plus *lalia*. Patients with **Tourette syndrome** sometimes have coprolalia.

The state of being mellow with a belly full of beer is to be **gambrinous**. The word comes from the name of **Gambrinus**, a mythical European champion of beer and joviality whose legend dates to the Middle Ages (Fig. 9.13).

The space between two teeth, usually the upper central incisors, is called a **diastema**, an adoption of the Greek *diastema*, or "space between."

When your arm "falls asleep" because of pressure on a nerve, the condition is called **obdormition**. The word, which can also simply mean being asleep, comes from the Latin *obdormire*, "to fall asleep."

To Avoid Offending Sensibilities

The extravagant delicacy of the refined class has given us many medical euphemisms, some with the intent of not offending, and some to render communication unintelligible to the uninitiated. For example, there are more than 100 euphemisms for the word **menstruation**, including the curse, being unwell, monthly blues, wallflower week, and little sister's here (Rawson, p. 181). The word **euphemism** comes from Greek *eu–*, meaning "good, well," and *pheme*, "utterance, speech." There are arguably so many health-related sensitive synonyms that euphemism might be considered a medical word.

One example of a medical euphemism is **stool specimen**. In Old English *stol* meant a "seat for one person." A later phrase was "close stool," describing a seat

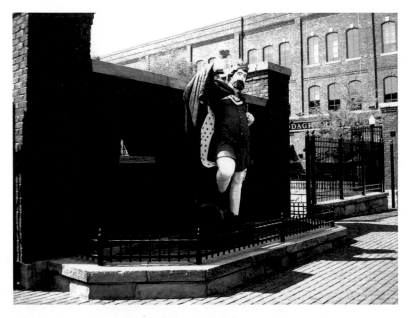

Fig. 9.13 Statue of King Gambrinus, in the Brewery District, Columbus, Ohio. Author: Columbusite. Creative Commons. https://commons.wikimedia.org/wiki/File:Statue_of_King_ Gambrinus,_Brewery_District,_Columbus,_Ohio.jpg

with an attached chamber pot in which one could make a fecal deposit during the night, and then close the lid until the contents could be emptied in the morning (Fig. 9.14). So, to be linguistically picky, sending the laboratory a stool specimen would seem to be sending part of a piece of furniture. The correct term would be **fecal specimen**.

Another euphemism for human feces is **bowel movement**, as digestive waste is produced in the act of defecation. In fact, there is some peristaltic movement of the large intestine that eventually culminates in the discharge of feces, sometimes incorrectly called stool, as described above. But to use the term bowel movement as a synonym for feces seems to say that you have expelled a piece of your intestine.

Did you ever wonder about the origin of the term **nonspecific urethritis**, a disease most commonly caused by *Chlamydia trachomatis*? It was created to differentiate the disorder from **specific urethritis**. And what is specific urethritis? The term, now archaic, was a euphemism for **gonorrhea**. Today **nonspecific urethritis** is more likely to be called **nongonococcal urethritis**, or **NGU**.

One euphemism still heard in obstetrical circles is the term **estimated date of confinement (EDC).** This, of course, is the projected date of a baby's birth, the "due date," calculated from the onset of the woman's last menstrual period. The quaint term "confinement" came from days when prolonged bed rest—a week of bed rest was once the standard—was one's reward for having a baby.

The term **disease** is, itself, a euphemism, coming from Old French *des–*, meaning "lack of," and *aise*, "ease." That is, when we consider the original meaning of

Fig. 9.14 Close stool, nineteenth century. Author: Flominator. Creative Commons. https://commons.wikimedia.org/wiki/File:Toilet_chair.jpg

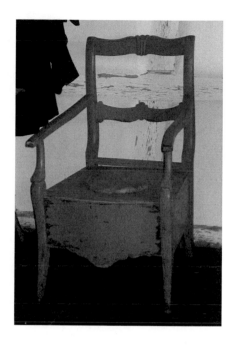

the root words, the person with a disease is not precisely *sick*; he or she is simply "without ease."

Acronyms

American physician Martin H. Fischer (1879–1962) writes, "Since the time of Hippocrates, our father, the aphorism has been the literary vehicle of the doctor" (Straus, p. 21). True, but more recently the doctor has embraced another literary vehicle: the **acronym**. The word **acronym** was coined in the 1940s from Greek *akron*, meaning "tip," and *onuma*, "name." An **acronym** is a word created from the first letters in a series of words. Often the acronymic word ceases to be a collection of first letters and becomes part of the language: examples or words making the leap from acronym to everyday word include laser (coming from "light amplification by stimulated emission of radiation") and zip code (the zip from "zone improvement plan").

An acronym differs from an **initialism** in that the acronym is pronounced as a word, such as AIDS (from acquired immunodeficiency disease) and an initialism is pronounced as a string of letters, such as HIV (from human immunodeficiency disease), pronounced H-I-V.

Here are a just a few current clinical acronyms:

- CREST: **c**alcinosis, **R**aynaud phenomenon, **e**sophageal dysmotility, **s**clerodactyly, and **t**elangiectasia

- HELLP syndrome: **h**emolysis, **e**levated **l**iver enzymes, **l**ow **p**latelets
- PANDAS: **p**ediatric **a**utoimmune **n**europsychiatric **d**isorders **a**ssociated with streptococcal infections
- PEEP: **p**ositive **e**nd-**e**xpiratory **p**ressure
- SLUD syndrome: **s**alivation, **l**acrimation, **u**rination, and **d**iarrhea

Even more recently we have seen the proliferation of acronymic research titles, some of them clearly tortured. Perhaps the reason for all the acronyms in the titles of research reports is that there is a positive correlation between the presence of an acronym in the title and the times an article is cited in the literature [15]. Here are a few creative acronymic research study titles:

- ALaCaRT: Effect of Laparoscopic-Assisted Resection vs Open Resection on Pathological Outcomes in Rectal Cancer
- BELT: Blacks and Exacerbations on LABA vs Tiotropium
- COPERNICUS: Carvedilol Prospective Randomized Cumulative Survey
- PROGRESS: Perindopril Protection Against Recurrent Stroke Study
- RALES: Randomized Aldactone Evaluation Study

Worth Saying Twice

As we end this section and this chapter, I want to alert you to the risks of contracting the **RAS syndrome**. This acronym **RAS** stands for **redundant acronym syndrome**. Manifestations of this malady are the use of phrases such as "PIN number," knowing full well that PIN stands for "personal identification number," and that saying PIN number is really saying "personal identification number *number*." In medicine, an example of the RAS syndrome is the term **ELISA test**, really saying "**enzyme-linked immunosorbent assay test**." Assay means test, hence the redundancy. This is almost as bad as saying "AIDS syndrome." Just as egregious is a phrase I used (purposely) in the first sentence of this paragraph: "the RAS syndrome," resulting in duplication of the word "syndrome."

References

1. Jamieson HC. Catechism in medical history. Can Med Assn J. 1943;48:148.
2. Karlen A. A capsule history of nostrums. Phys World. 1974;11(7):59.
3. Schartz H. Gabriel's palace: Jewish mystical tales. New York: Oxford; 1994, p. 58.
4. Roguin A. René Theophile Hyacinthe Laënnec (1781–1826): The man behind the stethoscope. Clin Med Res. 2006;4:230.
5. Cohen J. History lists: 9 bizarre baldness cures. Available at: http://www.history.com/news/history-lists/9-bizarre-baldness-cures
6. Altman LK. The doctor's world. The New York Times; November 30, 1982. Available at: http://topics.nytimes.com/top/news/health/columns/thedoctorsworld/index.html

7. Cheinisse L. Une cinquieme maladie eruptive: le megalerytheme epidemique. Sem Med. 1905;25:205.

8. Klein HO, Kaplinsky E. The Kochleffel syndrome. Arch Intern Med. 1983;143:135.

9. Derrick EH. "Q" fever, a new fever entity: clinical features, diagnosis, and laboratory investigation. Med J Aust. 1937;11:281.

10. Lerner AM. The abuse of paregoric in Detroit, Michigan (1956–1965). UNDOC Bulletin on Narcotics. 1966;3:13.

11. Aranson J. When I use a word. . . I mean it. BMJ. 1999;319(7215):972.

12. Morowitz HJ. How E. coli got its name. Hosp Prac. 1982;17(12):58.

13. Baker R. Epidemic: the past, present, and future of the diseases that made us. London: Vision Paperbacks; 2007. Available at: https://books.google.com/books?id=oWT0CQAAQBAJ&pg=PT40&lpg=PT40&dq=pustules+contain+a+perfect+smallpox+virus&source=bl&ots=rKBQ--TAWv&sig=QEyd8LD-CILCMGsZLvnjYfTX76o&hl=en&sa=X&ved=0ahUKEwi92PTGqnMAhUDWCYKHYvCBVcQ6AEIHDAA -

14. Bordenave G. Louis Pasteur (1822-1895). Microbes Infect. 2003;5:553.

15. Jacques TS, et al. The impact of article titles on citation hits: analysis of general and specialist medical journals. J Roy Soc Med. 2010; Available at: http://shr.sagepub.com/content/1/1/2.full

Chapter 10
Medical Words with Confusing and Controversial Origins

Among the joys of our amazing medical language are the occasional missteps, etymologic meanderings on the way to some of the words we use today. Some are simple misunderstandings. For example, the word **asphyxia** comes from Greek *a–*, meaning "without," and *sphyxis*, or "pulse." Although, granted, there is no pulse after death by suffocation, but we use the word **asphyxia** today to indicate interference with breathing, not arterial flow.

The source of our word **nerve** is the Greek *neuron*, meaning "bowstring," but Dirckx (p. 24) points out that the Greeks may have strung their bows with animal tendons, but certainly not with fragile nerve fibers.

The word **stupor** comes from the Latin *stupere*, meaning "to be astonished or struck senseless," although today the medical word indicates a state of numbness or lethargy. On the other hand, we also use the root in its original sense in **stupendous**, as in a "stupendous performance."

And there is the mistaken notion that the **guillotine** that beheaded many of the nobility during the French revolution in the late 1700s was the creation of French physician Joseph-Ignace Guillotin (1738–1814). The device was actually invented by a German harpsichord maker named Tobias Schmidt. Guillotin, speculated today to have opposed the death penalty, was guilty of simply advocating the guillotine as a more humane method of execution than hanging (Forsyth, p. 60) (Fig. 10.1).

Confusion can arise when body processes, structures, or fluids are mislabeled. For example, **Morton neuroma** is a misnomer; the cause of the foot pain is compression of the nerve as it passes under ligaments between the toe bones, usually between the third and fourth metatarsals, and not a tumor of the nerve. Another instance of muddled labeling is the term **synovia**, the name of the fluid that lubricates joints. Paracelsus (1493–1541) coined the term in 1520, from Greek *syn–*, "with," and *ovum*, "egg," suggesting a relationship of **synovial fluid** and egg white (Pepper, p. 36).

In medical etymology there are some epic misconceptions, terms describing things in ways about which we now know better. **Cholera** causes severe diarrhea, thought by the ancients to be a flow of Greek *khole*, or "bile." **Soroche**, another

© Springer International Publishing AG 2017
R.B. Taylor, *The Amazing Language of Medicine*,
DOI 10.1007/978-3-319-50328-8_10

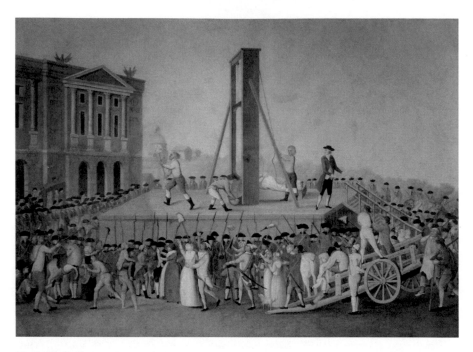

Fig. 10.1 Execution of Marie Antoinette in 1793 at the *Place de la Révolution*. Public Domain. https://commons.wikimedia.org/wiki/File:Exécution_de_Marie_Antoinette_le_16_octobre_1793.jpg

name for altitude sickness, is actually the Spanish word for the chemical element antimony; the disease was incorrectly thought be caused by the element, which is found high in the Andes Mountains.

No Air in the Artery

Names of body parts can be examples of mistaken word origins. The Greeks observed that after death, there was no liquid blood in the vessels that we now know carry blood. Believing the tubes were air ducts, they adopted the term *arteria*, meaning "windpipe," to describe them (Shipley, p. 290). It was not until 1628 that the circulation of blood was accurately described by British physician William Harvey (1578–1657).

Today, we know that an **artery** is a vessel that carries oxygenated blood from the heart. In fact, the presence of air in an artery would be an air **embolism**, the latter word coming from Greek *embolos*, meaning "wedge" or "plug." An air embolism can be a gaseous wedge that plugs an artery and causes an infarction or death.

A Legacy of Forbidden Fruit

We probably use the term **Adam's apple** more often than **laryngeal prominence** to describe the protrusion found at the angle of the thyroid cartilage anterior to the larynx (Fig. 10.2). Although present in both sexes, the **laryngeal prominence** is much larger in men, and thus is probably a male secondary sexual characteristic, related to deepening of the voice. The origin of the term Adam's apple, in any case, continues to be debated.

The most common theory is that the phrase Adam's apple comes from the ancient tale that a piece of forbidden fruit became stuck in the throat of Adam in the Garden of Eden (Evans, p. 9). Yet, according to Crabb, this story is absent from the Bible and other early Judeo-Christian teachings, and the apple is not specifically mentioned at all [1].

On the other hand, the whole thing could be a mistranslation. The name Adam came from the Hebrew word for "man," not unlikely since we are talking about the first male human. And the Hebrew terms for "bump" and "apple" are the same word (Haubrich, p. 5). So could an early term meaning "male bump" in Hebrew have been mistranslated to "Adam's apple"?

No Nasal Mucus at All

The Latin word *pituita* means "phlegm," and the **pituitary gland** is so named because of the mistaken belief that it is the source of mucus in the nose and throat (Dirckx, p. 66). Pepper (p. 47) traces the confusion to the time of Greek-Roman physician Claudius Galen (129–200), citing the belief that the oropharyngeal mucus came from the brain.

Then, according to Holmes et al., "Although Vesalius, perhaps the leading anatomist of all time, held a different view of the route taken by this mucus, the general idea was apparently accepted until the seventeenth century, when it was asserted by Schneider, and again by Richard Lower, that catarrhal secretions originated in the nasal passages, not in the brain" [2]. Thus, the pituitary gland gives us several essential hormones, but no nasal mucus at all.

Warty Growth, Thyme, and Soul

If you go to a fine French restaurant and order sweetbreads (*ris de veau*, in the language of Parisians), you will get a tasty dish, the **thymus gland** of a calf. A fleshy organ situated behind the sternum, the thymus gland plays an important immunologic role. **T lymphocytes**, or **T cells**, get their "T" from the name of the thymus

Fig. 10.2 The Adam's
apple, also known as the
laryngeal prominence.
Author: mysteriouskyn.
Creative Commons. https://
commons.wikimedia.org/
wiki/File:Male_neck.jpg

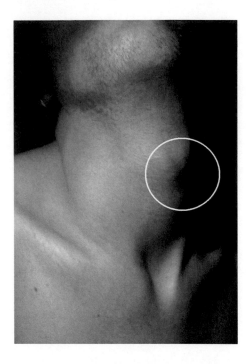

gland. The origin of the word **thymus**, however, has engendered the type of controversy that stirs the blood of word origin devotees.

Pepper (p. 36) tells that the thymus gland is named for its appearance, based on the Greek word *thymos*, meaning "warty growth." The gland is irregularly shaped and somewhat "bumpy" in appearance (Fig. 10.3). Perhaps, as postulated by Haubrich (p. 225), the term came from an alternative meaning of the Greek word *thymos*, the name of a member of the mint family of shrub that we today call thyme, as in the song "Parsley, Sage, Rosemary, and Thyme" by American singers Paul Simon and Art Garfunkel. Maybe the Greeks thought the gland resembled a bunch of thyme.

Yet another thought is that the gland was named for its location near the heart, because the homonymous Greek word *thymos* can also be translated as "soul," "desire," or "anger." Might the gland have thus been named by the Greeks because of its presumed connection to emotions?

Joe, the Fat Boy

At this point in the chapter, I turn from anatomy to diseases, beginning with a potentially fatal malady bearing a name rooted in literature.

The source of the **Pickwickian syndrome** represents an amusing misunderstanding and a tale that will break the heart of any serious poker player. The disease,

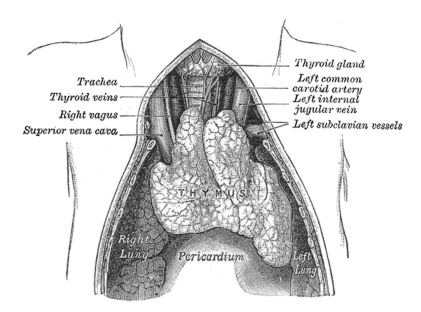

Fig. 10.3 The thymus. From: Gray H. *Anatomy of the Human Body*. Public Domain. https://commons.wikimedia.org/wiki/File:Gray1178.png

formally known as the **obesity hypoventilation syndrome**, is a condition of extremely obese persons who develop low blood oxygen levels and hypercapnia due to reduced respiratory effort. Excessive adiposity simply limits respiratory movement. One manifestation can be periods of uncontrollable sleepiness during the day. And that brings us to the Pickwick papers.

In 1837, British author Charles Dickens (1818–1870) published his first novel, *The Posthumous Papers of the Pickwick Club*. The book's main character was Samuel Pickwick, a benign and affluent man who was head of the Pickwick Club mentioned in the title. But the Pickwickian syndrome was not named for Samuel Pickwick.

One of the characters in the book was an immensely obese servant boy named Joe (Fig. 10.4). Joe was a voracious eater, and he tended to fall asleep while waiting tables. To quote Dickens:

"Damn that boy," said the old gentleman, "he's gone to sleep again."
"Very extraordinary boy, that," said Mr. Pickwick, "does he always sleep in this way?"
"Sleep!" said the old gentleman, "he's always asleep. Goes on errands fast asleep, and snores as he waits at table."
"How very odd!" said Mr. Pickwick.

The disease was given its eponymous name in 1956 by Burwell et al. in a paper describing a 51-year-old man carrying 260 pounds on his five-foot-five-inch frame. One evening at his weekly poker game, he had a full house—three aces and two kings—an almost sure winner. But he dropped off to sleep and failed to cash in his

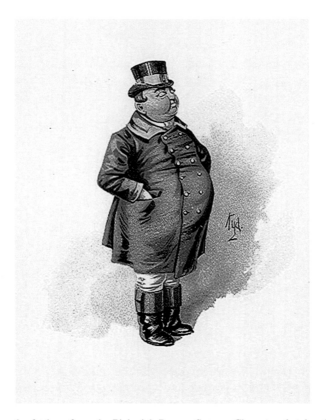

Fig. 10.4 Joe, the fat boy, from the Pickwick Papers. Source: Character sketches from Charles Dickens, Portrayed by Kyd. Public Domain. https://commons.wikimedia.org/wiki/File:The_Fat_Boy_1889_Dickens_The_Pickwick_Papers_character_by_Kyd_(Joseph_Clayton_Clarke).jpg

winning hand. Shortly thereafter he entered the hospital to treat his Pickwickian syndrome [3].

To be etymologically correct, the obesity hypoventilation syndrome should not be dubbed the Pickwickian syndrome, but rather the "fat boy syndrome," which would be politically incorrect, or perhaps simply "Joe's syndrome."

The Smug Sequences of Male-Dominated Thinking

The Greek word for **uterus** is *hystera*, and the word *hysterikos* described a malfunctioning uterus. According to Holt (p. 138), the Greeks believed that the psychological state of exaggerated excitement or emotion we now call **hysteria** originated in the womb. Perhaps that is why the disorder used to be called "mother-sick." Ciardi (p. 195) attributes this misperception to "the smug sequences of male-dominated thinking."

The word hysteria as a clinical diagnosis dates to at least the mid-seventeenth century. Today we have an entrenched misperception—**globus hystericus**—arising from an ancient belief that the "lump in the throat" felt with extreme emotion is actually the uterine fundus (Dirckx, p. 66).

Which Fire and Which Saint Anthony?

For starters, there are three diseases called **Saint Anthony's fire**, also known as **holy fire** or *ignis sacer*, and a host of individuals with the title of Saint Anthony. In the United States and Great Britain, the term Saint Anthony's fire is often used in connection with **erysipelas**, an acute infection with a skin rash, most often caused by beta-hemolytic group A streptococci. Bureau, writing in 1777, gave the name Saint Anthony's fire to erysipelas [4]. But the logic behind connecting the disease with the saint is murky.

In France and Germany, the term Saint Anthony's fire is more likely to indicate **ergotism**, the peripheral vasoconstriction that can result from excessive consumption of ergot, whether in bread made with contaminated rye fungus or overuse of ergot medication.

And in Italy, **herpes zoster**, the painful vesicles that can affect adults with incomplete immunity to the chickenpox virus, is sometimes called Saint Anthony's fire.

The title Saint Anthony has been given to at least dozen men, including Anthony the Younger, Anthony the Hermit, and Anthony of Rome. For our story, the most noteworthy are Saint Anthony the Great, also known as Saint Anthony of the Desert (Fig. 10.5), and Saint Anthony of Padua.

This brings us back to ergotism, which was common in the Middle Ages because consumption of bread made from wheat containing the *Claviceps purpurea* fungus resulted in burning sensations in the extremities, a feeling of "fire," sometimes followed by gangrene. Saint Anthony the Great (ca. 251–356) piously gave all his possessions to the poor and lived a monastic life (Fig. 10.5). Following his death, the Saint's remains were moved to various locations, eventually coming to rest in Dauphine, France. Then, in 1090, a wealthy French nobleman vowed to sacrifice all his fortune if only his son could be cured of ergotism. Following the young man's recovery, the father made good on his pledge, founding an order of monks that built hospitals to care for persons with ergotism. And Saint Anthony the Great also became the patron saint of those with ergotism.

But we must not forget Portuguese Franciscan Saint Anthony of Padua (1195–1231). He developed ergotism himself and died not long after. Relics of the Saint are preserved in the Basilica of Saint Anthony in Padua, and his name is also sometimes associated with ergot poisoning.

Fig. 10.5 Saint Anthony the Great, also called Saint Anthony of the Desert. Artist: Francisco de Zurbaran (1598–1664). Credit: Taragui. Public Domain. https://commons. wikimedia.org/wiki/ File:Anthony_Abbot_by_ Zurbaran.jpeg

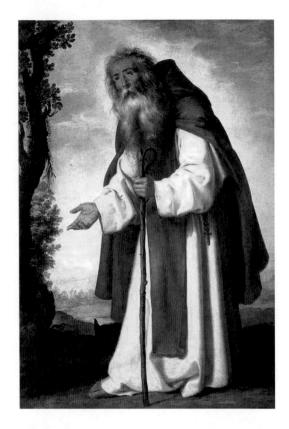

From a Linguistic Porcine Ancestor

Another disease from bygone days is **scrofula**, the term applied to tuberculosis of the lymph nodes of the neck, abscesses that can suppurate and form fistulas. The word scrofula comes from Latin *scrofa*, meaning "breeding sow," and spread of the tuberculosis infection to the skin is called **scrofuloderma**, with the suffix *–derma*, meaning "skin." The intriguing question is: How did this disease come to be named for an adult female hog?

Onions (p. 802) suggests that the lumpy cervical manifestations resemble the hog's back and then goes on to tell that breeding sows were thought to be subject to the disease. Pepper (p. 134) suggests "that the udders of old brood sows become lumpy, and the lumpy neck of a child with scrofula might be thought to resemble them." These are all good theories, but they give no clear answer to why the name of a cervical lymph node infection came from a porcine ancestor.

Tubercular cervical lymphadenitis once had another name, the **King's Evil**, or *morbus regius*. In medieval times, it was widely believed that the disease could be cured by the "royal touch." One notable example occurred in 1712, when Queen Anne touched the then-scrofulous child, Samuel Johnson, who would go on to live to age 75 and make huge contributions to English literature [5] (Fig. 10.6).

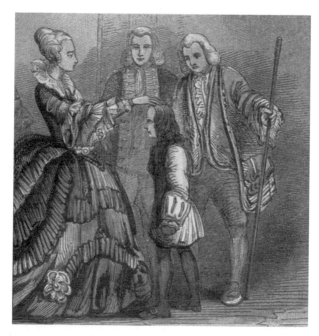

Fig. 10.6 Queen Anne touching Dr. Johnson, when a boy, to cure him of scrofula or the "King's Evil" (artist unknown). Public Domain. https://commons.wikimedia.org/wiki/File:Queen_Anne_"curing"_scrofula_by_touch.gif

When we look at the cause of scrofula, we find that it did not come from pigs, but was most often spread by the ingestion of milk from cows infected with tuberculosis. So maybe a better name for the disorder would be "vaccula," from *vacca*, Latin for "cow."

Oranges, Lemons, and Limes

As we wander through the garden of disease misnaming, we come to **scurvy**, the first disease to be recognized as caused by a dietary deficiency, as described in Chap. 3. The etymology is a little muddled, probably beginning with Latin *scorbutus*, meaning "scurvy," and then taking twists and turns through German, Old Norse, Dutch, and French. Haubrich (p. 202) points out: "Scurvy is somewhat of a misnomer.... It is an adjectival derivative of 'scurf,' a scaly exfoliation of the skin which is not a symptom of vitamin C deficiency as we now know it today."

To confuse the issue, scurvy has also been eponymously known as **Barlow's disease, Moeller's disease,** and **Cheadle's disease**. The first of these terms can be confusing: **Barlow syndrome** is used today as a synonym for **mitral valve prolapse**, and the two individuals named Barlow for whom the two entities are named are very different men who lived in different centuries.

Not Exactly the Seed of Life

The naming of **gonorrhea** should come under the heading: *Wow, did we ever get that wrong!*

The roots of the word gonorrhea are Greek *gonos*, meaning "semen, seed" and *rheos*, "flow." In the first century CE, Greek physician Aretaeus, who described many diseases and who gave diabetes it name, wrote about gonorrhea [6]. According to Pepper (p. 125), Aretaeus believed that the purulent discharge seen with gonorrhea was actually the result of penile paralysis causing the involuntary flow of semen.

In the 1800s, silver nitrate became a popular remedy for gonorrhea. Then, beginning at the turn of the century, American physician Albert Coombs Barnes (1872–1951) created **Argyrol**, a mild solution of **silver nitrate**, widely commercialized to treat gonorrhea. The brand name came from the Latin *argentum*, meaning "white metal, silver." Barnes became immensely wealthy, at least for his day, and began to collect art. The result is the Barnes Foundation Museum on Philadelphia's Benjamin Franklin Parkway, the home of scores of paintings by Renoir, Cezanne, Picasso, and many others. The therapy of gonorrhea has given the world a priceless art collection.

From the Bad Air

One disease that probably contributed to the fall of the Roman Empire was **malaria**, a mosquito-borne parasitic disease common in areas where mosquitoes breed in stagnant water. In the days of Roman emperors, there were marshes at many locations in Italy, including along the Tiber River (Fig. 10.7). The febrile disease came to be known as **Roman fever**.

The word malaria comes from Italian *mala*, meaning "bad," and *aria*, "air." It was believed that the disease was caused by **miasma**, or fetid air, a word coming from Latin *miasma*, meaning "noxious vapors." In fact, the air in swamps can be quite rank, but it does not cause the parasitic infection. The first use of the word malaria is credited to Italian physician Francisco Torti (1658–1741). The disease has also been called **marsh fever** and **ague**, the latter word coming from the Latin *acuta*, meaning "sharp," and suggesting the nature of the fever.

Malaria has existed in America since at least the fifteenth century, and at one time, malaria was endemic in every state of the United States except Alaska [7]. The disease continues to be a worldwide problem, afflicting some 200 million persons.

A Disease with Many Names

A mosquito-borne viral febrile disease, **dengue** was called **breakbone fever** by American physician Benjamin Rush (1746–1813) because of the severe joint pains that are characteristic symptoms. The original source of the word dengue may be the

Fig. 10.7 Tiber River in Rome. Author: MarkusMark. Public Domain. https://commons.wikimedia.org/wiki/File:001FiumeTevere.JPG

term *dinga*, part of *ka-dinga pepo*, a Swahili phrase describing disease caused by an evil spirit. In the 1820s, dengue came from Africa with slaves to the West Indies, where the name was influenced by the Spanish *dengue*, a word indicating "prudery," perhaps because of the primly stiff posture of those afflicted with bone and joint pains.

West Indian slaves with the disease were said to have **dandy fever**, a reference to the unusual gait of those afflicted. Along the way, **dengue fever** has also been called **bilious remitting fever, breakheart fever, Philippine fever**, and **Singapore hemorrhagic fever**.

Not Really Caused by Hay

Let's start with basics. **Hay fever** is not caused by hay, and there is no fever at all. In the tenth century, the Persian physician Rhazes (850–932) told of recurrent seasonal nasal congestion. The first clinical description of the affliction, at one time called **autumnal catarrh** (Bordley, p. 84), was by Italian Anatomist Leonardo Botallo (1519–1587). A British physician named Gordon erroneously named the disorder hay fever in 1829, presumably believing the symptoms were caused by newly mowed hay. In 1873, English physician Charles Harrison Blackley (1820–1900) demonstrated that the disease was caused by sensitivity to the pollens of grasses, trees, or weeds, some of which just happen to be prevalent during haying season.

The Original Spring Fever

Today what we call **spring fever** may be a sense of excitement experienced as winter ends and spring begins. Or the term may describe listlessness and sometimes a funky mood that comes as buds appear on the trees. There are various theories about the influence of serotonin, melatonin, and endorphins.

The etymologic curiosity is that just a few centuries ago, spring fever—the listless kind—was really scurvy, discussed above. After a long winter without vitamin-C-containing citrus fruits, by spring many persons suffered weakness, swollen joints, and perhaps even loose teeth. One author writes:

> I can also remember getting an orange in my Christmas stocking each year, a tradition continued by my parents from their youth, even though we usually had oranges in our house at the time. An orange would help keep the "Spring Disease" away, and in my parents' day oranges were far less common. An orange was a fitting "treat" and medicinal as well, at the beginning of winter [8].

Hypertension: Essential or Essential?

Look up the definition of **essential hypertension** and you will find some variation of the following: High blood pressure without a known cause. It is also referred to as **primary hypertension**. **Hypertension** with a known cause, such as chronic kidney disease, is called **secondary hypertension.**

But the original meaning of essential hypertension was something quite different. Just a few decades ago, high blood pressure, especially elevated systolic blood pressure, was not considered an important clinical finding. Physicians knew that, as persons aged, arteries became sclerotic, and they considered elevated blood pressure to be "essential" to propelling blood through the hardened arteries to vital organs. Thus the word "essential" in regard to blood pressure originally meant "necessary," rather than "of unidentified cause." In 1937, American cardiologist Paul Dudley White (1886–1973) wrote the following in his book titled *Heart Disease*:

> The treatment of hypertension itself is a difficult and almost hopeless task in the present state of our knowledge, and in fact for aught we know… the hypertension may be an important compensatory mechanism which should not be tampered with, even were it certain we could control it [9].

The Pharmaceutical Rx

Prior to the online communication of what medicine a patient should receive from the pharmacist, a written prescription began with the symbol **Rx**. The origin of this symbol is not entirely clear.

The Egyptian theory takes us to the time of the Egyptian physician Imhotep (ca. 2650–2600 BCE). According to legend, Horus, the benevolent son of Isis, had his eye gouged out by evil brother, Seth. The god of health, Thoth, replaced the lost vision, and the eye of Horus came to represent health and recovery from illness. The Rx symbol evolved as ancient Egyptian physicians and pharmacists combined various systems of weights and measures into an "eye of Horus" icon that very loosely resembles "Rx" (Fig. 10.8) [10].

On the other hand, because the ancient Romans often began prescriptions with a prayer to Jupiter, the **Rx symbol** may be a version of this god's alchemical symbol (Train, p. 51) (Fig. 10.9).

Sometimes the most likely theory is the correct one, and, despite the fanciful legends of Egyptian and Roman gods, the most likely source of the pharmaceutical symbol is that "Rx" is simply an abbreviation of the Latin word *recipe*, meaning "to take."

Fig. 10.8 Amulet with the Eye of Horus. Credit: From the excavations of Jacques de Morgan. Source: Marie-Lan Nguyen, 2005. Public Domain. https://commons.wikimedia.org/wiki/File:Eye_Horus_Louvre_Sb3566.jpg

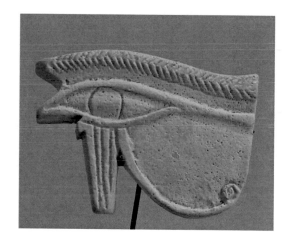

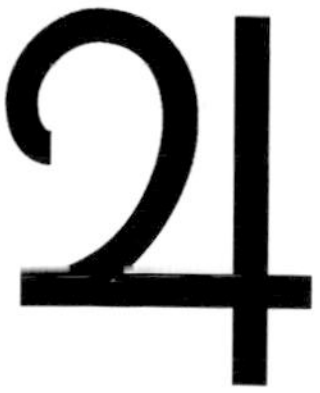

Fig. 10.9 Alchemical symbol of the planet Jupiter. This image shows the character U+2643 ♃ published by The Unicode Standard. Public Domain. https://commons.wikimedia.org/wiki/File:Jupiter_symbol.svg

The symbol Rx has spawned Hx (meaning history), Dx (diagnosis), and Tx (treatment), all unrelated to ancient Egyptians, Romans, and Latin word roots.

In Love at the Time

In 1864, German chemist Adolf von Baeyer (1835–1917) synthesized the first **barbiturate** by combining an ester derived from apples with urea from urine, and he named the compound, creating the new German word *Barbitursäure*, **barbituric acid** or simply **barbiturate**. There are several conflicting stories of how he chose this name.

Sensing the importance of what they had created, von Baeyer and his team toasted their as-yet-unnamed discovery in a tavern where, by chance, soldiers were celebrating the feast of Saint Barbara—the patron saint of artillerymen. During the imbibing and toasting, as the story goes, an artillery officer somehow decided to honor Saint Barbara, and he dubbed the new compound barbiturate (Fig. 10.10).

Another story (Youngson, p. 276) holds that the source of the urea in the new compound was the urine of a young beauty, a Munich waitress named Barbara. Li (p. 204) tells: "During his lectures, Baeyer used to say, 'At the time I was in love with a Miss Barbara. So I named my urea derivative barbituric acid.'"

Pepper (p. 100) has an entirely different theory. He suggests that word barbiturate is a thoughtfully constructed neologism, from the Latin *usnea barbata*, meaning "bearded moss," and *–urate*. I have searched and cannot find why von Baeyer would name his drug for what we call Spanish moss, unless it was an allusion to his own prominent beard.

Who Owns Aspirin?

The origin of the word **aspirin** is not controversial, but ownership of the word has a turbulent history. In 1898, German chemist Felix Hoffmann (1868–1946), working at the Friedrich Bayer Company, developed a new chemical which he found to have analgesic and antipyretic properties. He did so, at least in part, to help relieve the pain of his father's arthritis. The chemical name of the new compound became **acetylsalicylic acid**. The new drug was named brand-named **Aspirin** from *a–*, for "acetylation" and *spir*, from *Spiraea ulmaria*, the meadowsweet plant that is the source of salicylic acid. Bayer AG marketed Aspirin so energetically that it became the world's best-selling over-the-counter medication.

But Bayer Aspirin was to be a casualty of World War I. At the end of the conflict, the German company was declared "spoils of war," confiscated by the US government, and sold to Sterling Drugs for $5.3 million. Today the use of the term aspirin, without the modifier Bayer, is in the public domain, called a generic trademark.

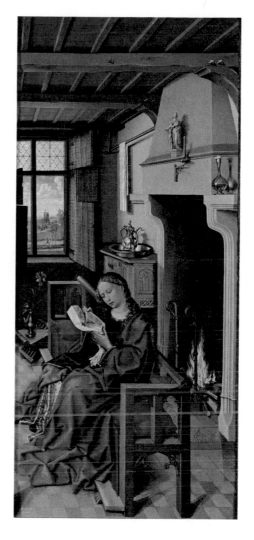

Fig. 10.10 Saint Barbara, from The Werl Altarpiece (1438) by Robert Campin. Public Domain. https://commons.wikimedia.org/wiki/File%3ARobert_Campin_015.jpg

The US trademark protection was lost when the US government seized the company as a war prize. Other products whose trade names have been genericized are escalator, thermos, cellophane, zipper, and heroin, the latter another trademark casualty of Bayer AG.

If It Has Wings, It's Not Medicine

Here we move from anatomy, diseases, and treatments to some general medical terms, starting with **caduceus**, from Doric Greek *kerukeion*, meaning a "herald's staff." The caduceus was the winged staff with two serpents twined around it and

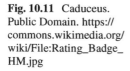

Fig. 10.11 Caduceus. Public Domain. https:// commons.wikimedia.org/ wiki/File:Rating_Badge_ HM.jpg

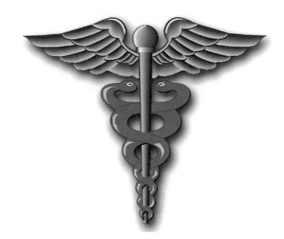

carried by Hermes, sometimes called "the messenger," as well as being the god of hospitality, diplomacy, travelers, shepherds, athletes, gamblers, liars, and thieves. In Roman times Hermes became Mercury, and from the Greek term came the Latin *caduceus*, the word used today. Today the caduceus is often used in the logos of various health care enterprises, notably hospitals.

This use of the caduceus in regard to medicine would all be just fine, except for one small fact. The true symbol of medicine is the **staff of Aesculapius**, with a single snake surrounding a wingless rod. The connection with medicine is that the snake, with its ability to shed its skin, was seen by the ancients as representing renewal and healing.

The confusion seems to have begun in 1851, when the US Army adopted the caduceus as a symbol for hospital stewards. Later the winged staff became part of the seal of the Army Medical Corps (Fig. 10.11). Today many consider the caduceus as representative of health care, but the true symbol of medicine is the Aesculapian rod with a single encircling snake (Haubrich, p. 34).

An Angel Dies

The word **patient** comes from Latin *patientem*, meaning "enduring suffering." On the way to the word we use today, the term spent time in Old French as *pacient* before becoming *pacyent* in Middle English. The term now means one who receives medical care and is only peripherally related to "being patient," describing one who endures a seemingly endless wait to see the doctor.

I hope that no one who is a student of the wonderful language of medicine ever refers to person receiving medical care as a **client**, fundamentally describing someone who engages the services of a lawyer, but now a term embraced by some commercial healthcare organizations. Nor should a suffering person be called a

customer. As quoted by Jackson: "I am reminded of the words of an anonymous surgeon: 'Every time a doctor calls a patient a *customer*, an angel dies'" [11].

Orthopedics and Pediatrics

In the year before his death, French physician Nicholas André (1658–1742), the first surgeon to correct scoliosis in a child, coined the word *orthopedia*, which he used as the title of a monograph on alleviating the deformities of children. In English the word is **orthopedic**, *orthos* meaning "straight, correct" in Greek. The original reference of the "ped" syllable in orthopedic was to children, just as **pediatrics** refers to the specialty focused on children.

But there is always an opportunity for confusion. In Greek, *pedon* means "ground." In Latin, *pes* means "foot." But none of this is related to orthopedics, even though many orthopedic specialists operate on the foot. Pepper (p. 147) points out that the name of the instrument for measuring the number of footsteps, the **pedometer**, was also once the name of a device used for measuring the height of children.

Menstruum, Menses, and Solvents

The words **menstruum** and **menses**, describing the monthly discharge of blood and discarded endometrial cells from the uterus of the nonpregnant female, come from a Latin word *mensis*, or "month."

But in medieval times the word *menstruum* also came to mean a **solvent**, in the sense that water is a solvent for sugar and turpentine dissolves oil-based paint. How did this change in the meaning of a straightforward term occur? Onions (p. 569) tells, "The development of the sense of 'solvent' in the medieval Latin arose from the alchemists' view of the transmutation of base metal into gold by a solvent liquid, which they compared to the development of the sperma in the womb by the agency of the menstrual blood." Thus the alchemists' appropriation of the *menstruum* term arose from a huge misunderstanding of the reproductive process.

Dutch physician Herman Boerhaave (1668–1738) had a somewhat different view: "Next we have an interesting explanation of the word menstruum.... The reason why this solvent was called a menstruum is because the chemists, in its application to the solvent, first used a moderate fire for a philosophical month, or 40 days; and hence called the solvent a *menstrual* solvent, and at length barely a menstruum" (Fig. 10.12) [12]. So, according to this theory, the alchemist's menstruum had to do with the calendar and nothing to do with periodic flow from the female uterus.

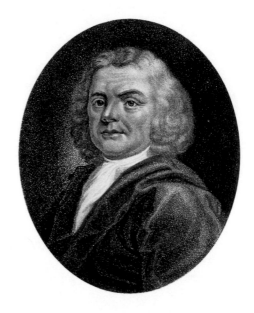

Fig. 10.12 Dutch physician Herman Boerhaave. Artist: J. Chapman. Public Domain. https://commons. wikimedia.org/wiki/ File:Herman_Boerhaave_ by_J_Champan.jpg

We no longer use menstruum and solvent as synonyms, but the somewhat confused pathway to their prior use gives insights into our linguistic history.

To Sheath and Protect

Penile sheaths to prevent disease and conception, what we now call **condoms**, have been around for centuries, and over the years have been made from oiled silk paper, animal intestines and gall bladders, animal horn, tortoise shells, and linen soaked in a chemical solution. An early description was written by Italian physician Gabriele Falloppio (1523–1562), and the device was later used by Italian adventurer and legendary womanizer Giacomo Casanova (1725–1798) to prevent his many mistresses from becoming pregnant.

The source of the word condom, however, is disputed. The word may have originated as a variation of the name French Cardinal Pierre de Gondi (1533–1616), protégé of Catherine de Medici and minister of Henry III of France in the sixteenth century, who developed waxed sheaths for his patrons, devices that came to be called *gondons* [13].

A popular, but unlikely, legend is that the item is named for a Dr. Condom, personal physician to Charles II of England (1630–1685), who provided sheaths for the royal penis [14].

Eatwell tells that the word condom may have come from the name of the village of Condom, in southwest France. Here, according to legend, local butchers used animal intestines to make penile sheaths [15]. As it happens, the village of Condom was on the Way of Saint James, the fabled route beginning in France and ending at the Cathedral of Santiago de Compostela in Galicia in northwest Spain. As the tale goes, the villagers sold their barrier devices to pilgrims traversing the route. Eventually some travelers shared these devices with friends at home, and the condom came to be called a **French letter** (Taylor, 2016, p. 107).

I am aware that all of the theories above have detractors, notably the inhabitants of the lovely town of Condom, and the answer may be as simple as that condom comes from the Latin word *condere*, "to sheath" [16].

Happy Birthday, Young Gaius Julius

Ask any young physician about the origin of the term **caesarean section,** and you will probably be told that the term goes back to the birth of young Gaius Julius Caesar in July, 100 BCE, through an incision in his mother's abdominal wall (Fig. 10.13). But this quaint tale is probably wrong.

One strong piece of evidence refuting the legend is that Caesar's mother, Aurelia Cotta, lived another 54 years after giving birth to the future Roman dictator. In those days, abdominal surgical extraction of a fetus was done only when the mother had died.

A more likely story is that the Caesar was a family name, and Ciardi (p. 54) describes the name of baby Gaius Julius Caesar as "signifying Gaius (given name) of the Julian clan (of Etruscan origin) of the family Caesar." Perhaps one of Gaius' ancestors had actually been born by "C-section." Note that the term caesarean comes from the Latin *cadere*, meaning "to cut."

Gould and Pyle have another entry into the etymologic sweepstakes. They suggest that the term caesarean comes from Latin *caesarise*, "head of hair," alluding to the thick head of hair of Gaius Julius at birth, or perhaps of some Caesar ancestor [17].

It was not until the sixteenth century that abdominal hysterotomy to facilitate childbirth was done on a living woman (Pepper, p. 170). And Gould and Pyle report that it was in the sixteenth century that Jane Seymour (1508–1537), destined to be the third wife of King Henry VIII, "was supposed to have been delivered of Edward VI, by caesarean section, the father, after the consultation of the physicians was announced to him, replying: 'Save the child by all means, for I shall be able to get mothers enough'" [17].

The Mad Atter

All who have read *Alice's Adventures in Wonderland*, written in 1865 by British author Lewis Carroll (1832–1898), know of the Mad Hatter (Fig. 10.14). Your parents or grandparents may have described someone acting oddly as being **mad as a hatter**. In fact, Alice and Carroll can be credited with popularizing the phrase. Although the term probably never appeared on a clinical record, there is a plausible and engaging medical theory behind its origin.

Fig. 10.13 Portrait of Gaius Julius Caesar, in British Museum. Author: Mark James Miller. Public Domain. https://commons.wikimedia.org/wiki/File:Portrait_of_Julius_Caesar_(color).jpg

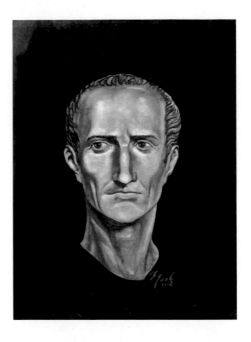

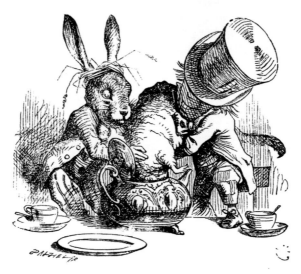

Fig. 10.14 The Mad Hatter and the Rabbit at tea. Author: John Tenniel (1820–1914). Public Domain. https://commons.wikimedia.org/wiki/File:Alice_par_John_Tenniel_27.png

Beginning in the eighteenth century, **mercury** was part of the process of making the felt used in hats. Daily exposure to the metal led to absorption and the development of **mercury poisoning** manifestations, which can include disturbed mental function. In the nineteenth century, a leading industry of the town of Danbury,

Connecticut was the manufacture of felt hats, and those involved sometimes developed a syndrome of uncontrollable tremors, a lurching gait, and mental aberrations that came to be called the **Danbury Shakes** [18].

All the above is medically correct, but probably not the origin of the term. The use of the phrase "mad as a hatter" was in common use before the advent of making felt hats (Morris, p. 360). And English author William Thackeray (1811–1863) used the phrase in his 1848 book *The History of Pendennis*, 17 years before Carroll penned *Alice*. Morris' theory is that hatter is derived from Anglo-Saxon *atter*, meaning "poison." "*Atter* is closely related to 'adder,' the venomous viper whose sting was thought to cause insanity" (Morris, p. 361).

Western, Southern, and Other Blots

The **Western blot** is an antibody detection test used in the diagnosis of human immunodeficiency virus (HIV) infection. The test, however, was neither developed in the west nor is it the product of research by anyone named West.

The test was named in 1981 by Burnette [19]. The name Western blot, perhaps selected with tongue in cheek, followed the **Southern blot** test. The **Western blot** originated in 1979 in Switzerland, definitely not the "West" by anyone's geographic reckoning. The name was simply a play on the previously developed Southern blot. The Southern blot technique had been eponymously named for its development in 1975 by English molecular biologist Edwin Southern (born 1938), while working at the University of Edinburgh (Haubrich, p. 247) (Fig. 10.15). There are now Northern

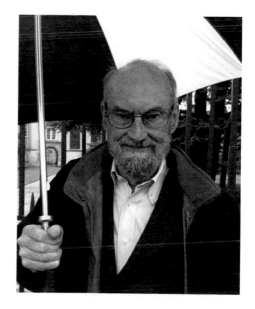

Fig. 10.15 Edwin M. Southern in 2012. Source: Gitschier J (2013) Problem Solved: An Interview with Sir Edwin Southern. PLoS Genet 9 (3): e1003344. Author: Jane Gitschier. Creative Commons. https://commons.wikimedia.org/wiki/File:Edwin_Mellor_Southern_-_journal.pgen.1003344.g001.png

blot, Eastern blot, and several other blot tests, all with geographic-sounding names with no eponymous significance.

The Last Entry in the Book

The previous paragraph was the book's **penultimate**, from Latin *penultimus*, or "next to last." This is the **terminal** entry, the word coming from the Latin *terminalis*, "pertaining to an end, final." The word terminal, of course, has a medical meaning, but here I use the word in the sense of coming to a close. I hope you have enjoyed the past ten chapters. I have certainly had fun researching and writing the tales. If you have a good word origin story, I would be happy to have you share it with me: taylorr@ohsu.edu. In the meantime, thank you for reading my book.

References

 1. Crabb G. Universal technological dictionary. Baldwin, Cradock, and Joy; 1823: "Pomum Ada'mi."
 2. Holmes RL et al. The pituitary gland: a comparative account. London: Cambridge University Press; 1974, p. 1.
 3. Burwell CS et al. Extreme obesity associated with alveolar hypoventilation; a Pickwickian syndrome. Am J Med. 1956;21:811.
 4. Bureau J. An essay on the erysipelas or that disorder commonly called St. Anthony's fire. London: J Johnson; 1777.
 5. Hitchings H. Dr. Johnson's dictionary: the book that defined the world. London: John Murray Publishers; 2006, p. 11.
 6. Tekiner H. Aretaeus of Cappadocia and his treatises on diseases. Turkish Neurosurg. 2015;25:508.
 7. History of malaria in the USA. Available at: http://dcmosquitosquad.com/history-of-malaria-in-the-usa/
 8. Janson P. When spring fever was a real disease. https://pauljanson.wordpress.com/2013/04/26/when-spring-fever-was-a-real-disease/
 9. White PD. Heart disease, 2nd Ed. New York: Macmillan; 1937, p. 326.
10. Green JR. Medical history for students. Springfield, Illinois: Charles C. Thomas; 1968, p. 13.
11. Jackson WC. In a word. JAMA. 1998;280:493.
12. Lloyd JU. Pharmaceutical preparations of plants. The Eclectic Med J. 1883;XLIII:203.
13. Collier A. The humble little condom: a history. Amherst, NY: Prometheus Books; 2007.
14. Bollet AJ. Medical history in medical terminology, part 2. Resid Staff Physician. 1999;45:60.
15. Eatwell PM. They eat horses, don't they? The truth about the French. New York: Thomas Dunne Books; 2014, p. 105. Available at: https://books.google.com/books?id=YMDCAwAAQBAJ&pg=PA105&lpg=PA105&dq=condom+french+village&source=bl&ots=9Ce0MTMBsF&sig=FhreDhHjX1R36T_FeQMJm-g6RVM&hl=en&sa=X&ved=0ahUKEwid5rfY7-HMAhVLNSYKHU2aA3I4ChDoAQgbMAA - v=onepage&q=condom french village&f=false
16. Amy JJ, et al. The condom: a turbulent history. Eur J Contracept Reprod Health Care. 2015;20:387.

17. Gould GM, Pyle WL. Anomalies and curiosities of medicine. Philadelphia: Saunders; 1901, p. 128. Available at: https://books.google.com/books?id=4k1rAAAAMAAJ&pg=PA128&lpg =PA128&dq=Save+the+child+by+all+means,+for+I+shall+be+able+to+get+mothers+enoug h&source=bl&ots=dlzFxclDn1&sig=0xBJf6rw32Rg7ClvpLBs-1guuwc&hl=en&sa=X&ved =0ahUKEwjbpPTD-uPMAhVHyyYKHZ25C6cQ6AEIHDAAvh]]

18. Mercury Workshop. Ohio Indoor Air Quality Coalition. Columbus OH: Ohio EPA; 2008, p. 23.

19. Burnette WH. Western blotting: electrophoretic transfer of proteins from sodium dodecyl sulfate—polyacrylamide gels to unmodified nitrocellulose and radiographic detection with antibody and radio-iodinated protein A. Analytical Biochem. 1981;112:195.

Acknowledgements

Recently I saw a roadside sign that read, "If you can read this, thank a teacher."

I hereby thank all my teachers in the Monongahela, PA public school system, at Bucknell University, and at Temple University School of Medicine who fostered my love of language, especially the language of medicine.

I am also grateful to colleagues and friends who, over the years, have tolerated my tendency to divert conversations by telling the curious origin of a word someone happened to use. This sort of pedantry must be truly annoying, but these kind persons put up with me, nevertheless. These patient individuals include: Charles (Chuck) Visokay, Joseph E. (Joe) Scherger, Peter A. Goodwin, Merle Pennington, John Kendall, William (Bill) Toffler, John Saultz, Scott Fields, Daniel J. Ostergaard, Robin Hull, Robert (Bob) Bomengen, Ray and Nancy Friedman, Tom Hoggard, Mary Burry, Ryuki Kassai, Takashi Yamada, Manabu Yoshimura, Michiyasu Yoshiara, Subra Seetharaman, Richard Colgan, Molly Osborne, Gary and Suzanne Bullock, Ben and Louise Jones, and E. Thomas (Tom) Deutsch.

I acknowledge with gratitude Coelleda O'Neil, who worked with me on a quarter-century's worth of books, as well as Margaret Moore and Michael Wilt of Springer Publishers who helped with the current book in many ways.

Thanks also to my wife, Anita D. Taylor, MA Ed, medical educator and author, who, through some 35 books and many published reports, has read every word I ever wrote or edited, and who didn't hesitate to ask, "Are you really sure you want to say that?"

© Springer International Publishing AG 2017
R.B. Taylor, *The Amazing Language of Medicine*,
DOI 10.1007/978-3-319-50328-8

Bibliography

This is a list of books recommended for the reader interested in the language of medicine and the origins of the terms we use today.

Ackerknecht EH. *History and Geography of the Most Important Diseases*. New York: Hafner; 1972.

Adler RE. *Medical Firsts: From Hippocrates to the Human Genome*. New York: Wiley; 2004.

Bean RB, Bean WB. *Aphorisms by Sir William Osler*. New York: Henry Schuman; 1950.

Bollett AJ. *Plagues and Poxes: The Impact of Human History on Epidemic Disease*. New York: Demos; 2004.

Bordley J, Harvey AM. *Two Centuries of American Medicine*. Philadelphia: Saunders; 1976.

Brallier JM. *Medical Wit and Wisdom*. Philadelphia: Running Press; 1994.

Breighton P, Breighton G. *The Man Behind the Syndrome*. Heidelberg: Springer-Verlag; 1986.

Cartwright FF. *Disease and History: The Influence of Disease in Shaping the Great Events of History*. New York: Crowell; 1972.

Ciardi J. *A Browser's Dictionary*. New York: Harper & Row; 1980.

Colgan R. *Advice to the Healer: On the Art of Caring*. New York: Springer; 2013.

Dirckx JH. *The Language of Medicine: Its Evolution, Structure, and Dynamics*, 2nd edition. New York: Praeger; 1983.

Durham RH. *Encyclopedia of Medical Syndromes*. New York: Harper and Brothers; 1960.

Evans B, Evans C. *A Dictionary of Contemporary American Usage*. New York: Random House; 1957.

Evans IH. *Brewer's Dictionary of Phrase and Fable*. New York: Harper & Row; 1970.

Fabing HJ, Marr R, editors. *Fischerisms, Being a Sheaf of Sundry and Diverse Utterances Culled from The Lectures of Martin H. Fischer, Professor of Physiology in the University of Cincinnati*. Springfield: Illinois: Charles C. Thomas; 1937.

Firkin BG, Whitworth JA. *Dictionary of Medical Eponyms*. Park Ridge NJ: Parthenon; 1987.

Forsyth M. *The Etmyologicon: A Circular Stroll through the Hidden Connections of the English Language*. New York: Berkley Books; 2011.

Fortuine R. *The Words of Medicine: Sources, Meanings, and Delights*. Springfield, Illinois: Charles C. Thomas; 2001.

Garrison FH. *History of Medicine*, 4th edition. Philadelphia: Saunders; 1929.

Gershen BJ. *Word Rounds*. Glen Echo, Maryland: Flower Valley Press; 2001.

Gordon R. *The Alarming History of Medicine: Amusing Anecdotes from Hippocrates to Heart Transplants*. New York: St. Martin's, Griffin; 1993.

Haubrich WS. *Medical Meanings: A Glossary of Word Origins*. Philadelphia: American College of Physicians; 1997.

Hendrickson R. *The Literary Life and other Curiosities*. New York: Viking; 1981.

© Springer International Publishing AG 2017
R.B. Taylor, *The Amazing Language of Medicine*,
DOI 10.1007/978-3-319-50328-8

Holt AH. *Phrase and Word Origins: A Study of Familiar Expressions.* New York: Dover; 1961.
Huth EJ, Murray TJ. *Medicine in Quotations: A View of Health and Disease through the Ages.* Philadelphia: American College of Physicians; 2006.
Inglis B. *A History of Medicine.* New York: World; 1965.
Jablonski S. *Jablonski's Dictionary of Syndromes and Eponymic Diseases,* 2nd ed. Malabar FL: Krieger; 1991.
Li JJ. *Laughing Gas, Viagra, and Lipitor: The Human Stories behind the Drugs We Use.* New York: Oxford; 2006.
Lindsay JA. *Medical Axioms, Aphorisms, and Clinical Memoranda.* London: H.K. Lewis Co.; 1923.
Magalini SI, Scrascia E. *Dictionary of Medical Syndromes,* 2nd edition. Philadelphia: Lippincott; 1981.
Major RH. *Disease and Destiny.* New York: Appleton-Century; 1936.
Maleska ET. *A Pleasure in Words.* New York: Fireside Books; 1981.
Martí-Ibáñez F. *A Prelude to Medical History.* New York: MD Publications; 1961.
Mayo CH, Mayo WJ. *Aphorisms of Dr. Charles Horace Mayo and Dr. William James Mayo.* Willius FA, editor. Rochester MN: Mayo Foundation for Medical Education and Research; 1988.
McDonald P. *Oxford Dictionary of Medical Quotations.* New York: Oxford University Press; 2004.
Meyers MA. *Happy Accidents.* New York: Arcade Books; 2007.
Morris W, Morris M. *Morris Dictionary of Word and Phrase Origins.* New York: Harper & Row; 1971.
Oldstone MBA. *Viruses, Plagues, and History.* New York: Oxford University Press; 1998.
Onions CT. *The Oxford Dictionary of English Etymology.* Oxford: Clarendon Press; 1979.
Online Etymology Dictionary. Available at: http://www.etymonline.com
Osler W. *Aequanimitas with other Addresses.* Philadelphia: Blakiston; 1906.
Oxford English Dictionary. Available at: www.oed.com
Paulman P, Taylor RB. *Family Medicine: Principles and Practice,* 7th edition. New York: Springer; 2016.
Penfield W. *The Torch.* Boston: Little, Brown and Co.; 1960.
Pepper OHP. *Medical Etymology.* Philadelphia: Saunders; 1949. Available at: https://catalog.hathitrust.org/Record/002077659
Porter R. *The Greatest Benefit to Mankind.* New York: Norton; 1997.
Porter R. *Blood and Guts: A Short History of Medicine.* New York: Norton; 2004.
Rapport S, Wright H. *Great Adventures in Medicine.* New York: Dial Press; 1952.
Rawson H. *A Dictionary of Euphemisms and other Doubletalk.* New York: Crown; 1981.
Sebastian A. *The Dictionary of the History of Medicine.* New York: Parthenon; 1999.
Shipley JT. *Dictionary of Word Origins.* New York: Philosophical Library; 1945.
Shryock RH. *Medicine and Society in America: 1660–1860.* Ithaca, New York: Cornell University Press; 1960.
Skinner HA. *The Origins of Medical Terms.* Baltimore: Williams & Wilkins; 1949.
Silverman ME, Murray TJ, Bryan CS. *The Quotable Osler.* Philadelphia: American College of Physicians; 2003.
Strauss MB. *Familiar Medical Quotations.* Boston: Little, Brown; 1968.
Taylor RB. *Medical Writing: A Guide for Clinicians, Educators, and Researchers,* 2nd edition. New York: Springer; 2011.
Taylor RB. *White Coat Tales: Medicine's Heroes, Heritage and Misadventures,* 2nd edition. New York: Springer; 2016.
Train J. *Remarkable Words with Astonishing Origins.* New York: Charles N. Potter; 1980.
Weisse AB. *Medical Odysseys: The Different and Sometimes Unexpected Pathways to Twentieth-Century Medical Discoveries.* New Brunswick, New Jersey: Rutgers University Press; 1991.
Youngson RM. *Medical Curiosities.* London: Robinson Publishing; 1999.

Index

A

Abattoir fever, 186
Abdomen, 4
Abernathy biscuit, 126
Abernathy, J., 126
Academe, 11
Academia, 9–11
Academic, 9–11
Academus, 10, 11
Acctabulum, 1, 2
Achilles tendon, 2, 3
ACHOO syndrome, 114
Acid, 30–31, 34
Acronym, 173, 193–194
Acute necrotizing ulcerative gingivitis, 90
Adam's apple, 199, 200
Adder, 217
Addison disease, 127
Addison, T., 127
Addisonian anemia, 127
Addisonian crisis, 127
Addisonism, 127
Adonis, 14, 16
Aesculapian rod, 212
Aesculapius, 9, 16–17
Agar, 5, 68–69
Agoraphobia, 159, 187
Ague, 206
Air embolism, 198
Alcohol, 63
Alice in Wonderland syndrome, 138
Alice's Adventures in Wonderland, 138, 215
Allergic salute, 105
Alopecia, 183, 184
Alopecia areata, 183, 184
Alopecia totalis, 183

Alzheimer disease, 133
Alzheimer patients, 67
Alzheimer, A., 133
AMBER alert, 114
Ambidextrous, 149
Ambivalence, 160
Ammonia (NH3), 82
Amok, 67–68
Amuck, 67–68
Amygdalin (Laetrile), 83
Amyloid, 111
Anaphylaxis, 164
Anchovy sauce stools, 99
Androgenic alopecia, 124, 183
Androgynous, 15
Android, 111
Anechoic, 112
Anesthesia, 150, 158
An evening with Venus, 12
Angina pectoris, 154–155
Anisosterixis, 179
Antecubital fossa, 180
Anthrax, 108, 109
Antibiotic, 168, 173, 188
Antitoxin, 179
Aphrodisiac, 14
Aphrodite, 9, 14–16, 20
Apollo, 9, 11, 12, 16, 22, 23
Apollo disease, 11
Apollo space program, 11
Apothecary, 54
Appendicitis, 159–160
Arenaviridae, 80
Aretaeus, 206
Aretaeus the Cappadocian, 36
Argyrol, 206

© Springer International Publishing AG 2017
R.B. Taylor, *The Amazing Language of Medicine*,
DOI 10.1007/978-3-319-50328-8